rain forest wisdom
what gorillas tell us about ourselves

rain forest wisdom
what gorillas tell us about ourselves

by Andrew Y. Grant

illustrated by Zachary Horvath

TATRA PRESS LLC

TATRA PRESS

Croton-on-Hudson, New York

2013

*I dedicate this book to all gorillas, to my friends,
and my family group, especially Christan, Chad, Shannon, Jenny and
my grandchildren Eva, Anthony, Lane, Charlie, Romi, and Flavin.*
—Andrew Y. Grant

RAIN FOREST WISDOM: What Gorillas Tell Us About Ourselves

Copyright © by Andrew Y. Grant 2013.
Illustrations Copyright © by Zachary Horvath 2013.

Library of Congress Control Number: 2013947660
ISBN 13: 978-0981932194
Printed in the United States of America.

For author, publisher or special bulk-order enquiries:
Chris Sulavik
Tatra Press LLC
4 Park Trail
Croton-on-Hudson, NY 10520
Email: tatrapress@gmail.com

Book design and text composed by Stephanie Bart-Horvath.

Publisher's Note: Much of the material in this book originally
appeared in *Nearly Human: The Gorilla's Guide to Good Living*
(Tatra Press, 2007)

www.tatrapress.com

Contents

acknowledgments

I'd like to express my deep appreciation not only to my family, but also to my publisher, Christopher Sulavik, for helping to shepherd this project from concept to book. His encouragement and support are greatly appreciated.

A special acknowledgment goes to Geoff Howard-Spink, whose enthusiasm and friendship were vital.

I am grateful for the work of the many talented and devoted people in this field who laid the groundwork for gorilla conservation, and I would like to acknowledge them, particularly: Dr. Dian Fossey, Dr. George Schaller, Dr. Jane Goodall, Dr. Penny Patterson, Dr. David Watts, Dr. Alice Honig, Dr. Kelly Stewart, Dr. Alexander Harcourt, Dr. Allison Fletcher, Dr. Juichi Yamagiwa, Dr. Alan Dixon,

Bob Wiese, Carmi Penny, Yvonne of San Diego and the Consortium for the Reproduction of Miles, Christina Simmons and Dr. Martha Robbins.

Many thanks to the Zoological Society Endangered Species, especially Director Doug Myers, Ted Molter, Andy Philips, and Peggy Blessing, for their support and input. To Zachary Horvath, whose illustrations made the book come alive, and to Stephanie Bart-Horvath, who designed the book, thank you, and thanks to Erin Patterson for her editing.

I hope that when my grandchildren are old enough, they will have an opportunity to see gorillas in the wild.

introduction

Through the decades I have worked with zoos, I have long been fascinated by the wonders of all animals. I've taken a special interest in endangered species and have been fortunate to contribute to efforts protecting them.

But, of all endangered species, it's impossible to ignore one: the gorilla.

Although all animals are indeed "created equal," the fact is that we humans, when visiting zoos, tend to hang out near the primate enclosures—especially those with gorillas inside. Why? For myriad reasons, I suppose. Their size, their grace, their curiosity, their power. But mostly, I believe, there exists a search for a connection between people and gorillas. I've seen this countless times, this special interspecies mutual

9

appreciation. People try, in their quirky human ways, to bond with the gorillas. Gorillas, in turn, can connect with the fortunate among us.

Clearly, something profound happens when we and one of our closest relatives—the gorilla—share cognitions. Despite all our differences, we see striking similarities. Through our mutual suspicions, we sense an odd kinship. Something happens, surely, and I suppose it's different with different people. Some readers may embrace these similarities with interest and, hopefully, a knowing smile. Others may balk. Yet no one can ignore the overarching question that beckons when staring eye-to-eye with this amazing creature: *How gorilla are we?* And perhaps more important... *What do gorillas tell us about ourselves...about being human?*

I wrote this book to help make finding the answer a bit easier; to help come closer to understanding the wonders of this proud animal; and, possibly, to help us understand ourselves a little better.

I also endeavor to share what I believe are some of the most fascinating and important findings of hundreds of brilliant and tireless primatologists, anthropologists, and others. I cast a particularly bright light on the rich and admirable research and findings surrounding the mountain gorillas of the Virunga Mountains in equatorial Africa, where many dedicated scientists, including pioneers George Schaller and Dian Fossey, have been studying this captivating animal for more than four decades.

And, finally, there's the motivation that this book, to some degree, may help its subject—the gorilla. If *Rain Forest Wisdom* can help raise public awareness of the gorilla, my hope is that it will also prompt conservation efforts and involvement in helping to protect this endangered species, as well as others. In a way, the gorilla provides us with vital clues to our own natures, as well as our successes and failures as a species.

I do believe that in many ways, the actions needed to save the gorilla are the same steps we need to take to save ourselves.

Andrew Y. Grant
Santa Barbara, California, 2013

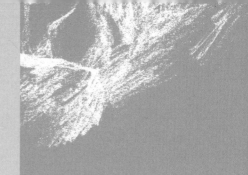

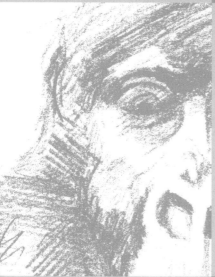

note to reader

There are references throughout this book to the various gorilla subspecies. For details on nomenclature, taxonomy and distinguishing characteristics of these subspecies, please consult chapter six, gorilla nomenclature and species characteristics.

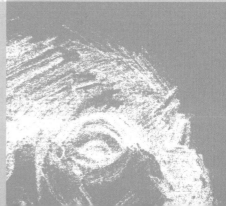

chapter one

growing up

The nostalgia of childhood...cutting through the neighbor's yard to meet friends, coming home any time, as long as it's before dark. Times have changed, and so, too, have childhoods, with fences going up restricting kids from the freedoms we remember.

Field studies tell us that young gorillas are given the space to explore, and that they need that space to be tireless learners and spirited playmates. They jump into situations with little or no prodding or guidance by parents. A good hunch is that there's some connection between the confidence of young gorillas and an upbringing filled with the freedom to grow at one's own pace.

But growing up is never easy, especially in the wild. Roughly half of the wild mountain gorilla population does not survive beyond the age of six. Young gorillas die early for a variety of reasons: they fall from trees, are attacked by predators, succumb to viruses, stillbirths, and poachers. There are still darker fates. Some mountain gorilla infant deaths are caused by infanticide perpetrated by males in order to "acquire" their mother, typically after she emigrates into a group with a child in tow.

Survivors are raised in a stable group, with loyal elders and an assemblage of kin, including half-siblings and even unrelated group members. By the time they can walk, most young gorillas have already absorbed—often through play—adult-like traits, behaviors and skills.

Mastering these skills doesn't come through boot-camp discipline and training. It comes from learning with others. Together, gorillas learn everything from splitting a stem and removing the pith, to nest building, and grooming.

This chapter takes a close look at a very, *very* traditional upbringing that, in some ways, can seem strangely progressive to those who consider some parenting conventions.

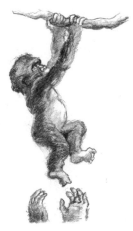

from zero to three: high-octane learners

In the first few months, gorilla babies seem quite human. Soon after birth, infants cling to their mother's chest hairs. The mother shows the newborn to group members, who touch and sniff at their "oohs" and "ahhs".

With their little ones attached, mothers literally carry (or, rather, lumber) on with their lives. They first carry infants under the chest with one arm and hobble on three limbs. Eventually, babies hitch rides on their mothers' backs. Slowly, very slowly, the mothers resume some semblance of life as it was before kids.

"The adult world is being separated from the child's world, and more children are feeling that childhood is a strange place. Just a generation ago, parents spent much more time including children in the everyday activities of their lives, which promotes confidence and a sense of independence."

—Eileen Hayes, Parenting Advisor, National Society for the Prevention of Cruelty to Children

birth in the wild

Observations of gorilla births in the wild are extremely rare, but anthropologist Kelly Stewart saw one in Rwanda on December 3, 1975. She wrote:

> *It was short (a couple of minutes), unaided, and didn't appear that painful. The mother receded from her group of 12 members, who clustered around her when she went into labor in thick vegetation. She gave birth while squatting, then licked the newborn, chewed the placenta. Soon after birth, the infant was cleaned of mucus, and held closely to the mother's chest—even*

being gingerly groomed by the mother's index finger. The newborn was as white as "polished alabaster," but the skin later turned pink. The mother supported the infant with her arm— her hand supporting the head and snuggled and rocked. When the newborn squealed, the mother responded with a soothing belch vocalization, then nestled it to her chest.

From six months on, infants gain skills at a swift clip. Primatologist George Schaller observed an infant, as young as eight months, attempting to build his own nest. Infants under the age of two craftily completed ground nests and also begin the far trickier task of building tree nests. By two years old, they are learning tactile and visual gestures, primarily for play and eating. One study even described two-year-old gorillas moving to break up fights between adult males.

Feeding progresses, too, so that by the age of three, mealtime is mainly self-service. Most three-year-olds have already mastered basic food processing techniques—splicing stems to reveal the preferred pith inside, stripping leaves

> Observations of gorilla births in the wild are
> extremely rare.

from vines, and eating stinging nettle or thistle—according to Richard Byrne, of the Scottish Primate Research Group and St Andrews University, who has studied how infants and juveniles process foods. Byrne found that mountain gorillas learn multi-step food processing through "individual exploration," which involves separating the preferred plant parts from non-nutritious, indigestible or even dangerous parts. They also learn how to gather fruit and to distinguish ripe from unripe fruits.

young mediators

In a study by Pascale Sicotte, more than 40 percent of all bust-ups between fighting adult male mountain gorillas are made by gorillas between the ages of two to six. A typical gorilla referee will run between the battling males and screech in a high-pitched voice used only in this situation. Referee gorillas cling to one of the battling male's chests, and might even be carried around for a few paces. These "interpositions" were not directed at any one male, and no interfering animal was hurt or attacked in these episodes. Sicotte even observed gorillas younger than two years old making vocalizations as their mothers mediated arguments among other members—though it was unclear to her whether these vocalizations were attempts at refereeing or rather responses to a mother's alarmed state.

By age three, gorillas have already mastered most of the complex food-prepping skills, like separating pith from stems and eating nettles without getting stung, according to primate researcher Richard Byrne.

old-school ties

Gorillas as young as two or three months old start reaching out to others. Because the mother is usually in the silverback's vicinity, it is the silverback (the principal of a group) that the infant gets to know first. Older infants (around the age of three) tend to spend more time near the silverback than do older members of the group.

Interestingly, orphans tend to have unusually close relationships with the silverback throughout their childhoods,

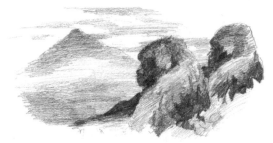

grooming him more than they groom others. It is thought that creating a bond with a silverback might provide a safer fate for an orphan than creating one with a mother substitute (who might transfer into a strange, new group).

Even at a young age, the benefits of getting along with the silverback are clearly evident, but relationships with other group members are crucial, too. These relationships create options for play and companionship. Later, these childhood relationships often evolve into important social alliances, which, ultimately, form a solid political base gorillas will need as they mature. Consider how young males, for example, pick up the art of protecting the group as "sentries" from older males, an important rung on the group's hierarchical ladder. Likewise, females observe the importance of grooming by watching their mothers, from whom they also learn the importance of keeping relations with the silverback strong.

what is family?

Gorilla groups are referred to as "groups," not "families". Though most, or even all, may be related, the groups change constantly, and can be composed of a jumble of closely related, remotely related or completely unrelated members. They are almost always led by a silverback who will dictate to the group—until he dies or is replaced by a successor, often his son (especially in mountain gorilla groups). Populations within groups change by the addition of new members through births, or migration either into or out of the group.

While a typical infant will spend at least the first few years with its mother and father, this "nuclear" arrangement obviously alters if the mother leaves the group (which is the case with the majority of females) or if the father dies. When a mother and infant join a new group, they must learn to form new ties quickly with non-kin or unrelated adults. Single mothers—and their kids—can face uphill struggles in creating such bonds with members of a new host group.

For gorillas, the larger the groups (generally), the better. More offspring means greater opportunities for all younger members to learn survival skills more quickly. Gorillas with older siblings and peers tend to break bonds of proximity and contact with adults earlier than those without older siblings and peers. Interestingly, during play, infants prefer to be around juveniles, but at rest, they prefer to be around other infants.

While siblings play an important role, bonds with the mother persist long after the mother is needed for milk or constant vigilance. Even at the age of four, gorillas can still have strong ties with their mothers, either as a source of protection and social support (such as acting as a trusted ally in a dispute with another group member) or as an important mentor in securing strong relationships and kinships.

The closeness between gorilla mothers and their young says a lot about the importance of the connections we make with our children during their formative years. "Nurturing mutual respect between parent and child helps children to socialize with peers and adults," says Eileen Hayes, author and parenting advisor for the National Society for the Prevention of Cruelty to Children (UK). "Most parents don't realize that kids actually like taking part in adult activities—like picking up, or dusting, or loading the washing machine. It makes them feel like part of the family. Mutual respect also comes by speaking to children with the patience and politeness that you show when speaking with a friend," says Hayes. "Ordering children around abruptly and rudely will only show the child that rude manners are acceptable, and is another way of excluding them and eroding mutual respect," she added.

the importance of play

Play is a sign of well-being, a platform for learning to communicate, a chance to improve coordination, and to assert independence. Although adult gorillas can accommodate play, they don't initiate it. There are exceptions, however. Mothers tickle infants and sometimes roll on the ground with them. Some silverbacks have been observed playing with infants.

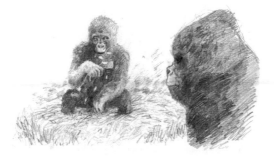

Typically, active and prolonged play among gorillas starts when the infant is about five months old and begins to taper off around the age of six years. Primatologist George Schaller noted that gorillas might play any time of day, but that it is typical for infants and juveniles to take off on their own and play after midday rests.

After gorillas hit puberty, play is rare. Young and older adults tolerate play around them—and on top of them—but are seldom seen initiating or taking part in play.

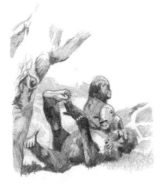

ROLE PLAY Roleplay offers younger gorillas the chance to practice skills they need later on, such as jumping, swinging, and somersaulting. It also lets them stretch the boundaries of communication in a non-threatening environment, such as trying out vocalizations of other group members or non-vocal forms of communication (i.e., tactile, auditory, and visual signals). Through role play, they learn to gauge the effect of these new behaviors on others.

LONE PLAY Examples of lone play include: climbing, swinging from vines, walking on fallen trees, hitting vegetation, tumbling, jumping, pulling limbs, sliding down vines, doing somersaults, and running back and forth with hands in exaggerated gestures. About half of primatologist George Schaller's observations were of gorillas playing alone. An usually "human" moment of play he encountered was of a gorilla infant placing a huge leaf on its head and standing motionless—in the same way a child may disguise himself with a paper bag.

Allison Fletcher, a researcher of gorilla social development, found that lone play in mountain gorillas peaks by the time they are 18 months old. At this stage, some infants might engage in lone play for periods up to nine minutes an hour. "[Infants] like to play with leaves, swirl and twirl their bodies, and roll in the vegetation," says Fletcher.

As the infant ages, lone play steadily decreases until it has almost disappeared by the age of 30 months.

SOCIAL PLAY Social play can involve wrestling, chasing one another, playing king-of-the-mountain, follow-the-leader, and even doing the conga. Sometimes youngsters wave their hands slowly over their heads while facing or approaching one another.

Play can also be a practice ground for asserting dominance and communicating subordination or passivity. Young gorillas overwhelmed by rough play, for example, do what's called the "submissive crouch," which might be compared to their human cousins crying "Uncle!" The submissive crouch is a surrender gesture and is the opposite of the threat gesture used by young gorillas when playing. When they play, young gorillas practice elements of dominant behavior: direct eye contact, lip tucking, standing on two legs, walking with stiff legs, strutting about, and chest beating. Young males try out menacing facial expressions like the "threat face" in which they open their mouths wide and display their teeth.

Playing infants have also been observed nipping softly at the nape of the neck, like the "mock biting" of mothers.

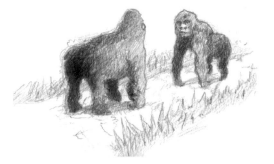

Young females spend time near mothers with infants, preparing for their future role in adult gorilla society.

Another adult domain—reproduction—is even explored by the young through play. Infants as young as around two years old start what's called "play copulations."

learning through play

Simone Pika of the Max Planck Institute for Evolutionary Anthropology in Leipzig, Germany, found that captive lowland gorillas aged one to six used 33 distinctive gestures. Interestingly, the three- and four-year-olds used more gestures than the five- and six-year-olds. All 33 gestures were used in the context of play but less than half were used while traveling, suggesting that gorillas use play to try out new gestures and communication strategies.

leaving the nest

When gorillas reach puberty, adult pressures escalate. The "teen" years, even among gorillas, are awkward for the entire group. During this stage, young males assert themselves, sometimes even competing with the silverback for access to females. Males either remain group members as subordinates to the silverback, or they leave. Childhood, for the gorilla, ends on one message: be my ally or leave.

Adolescent males receive the most aggression from the silverback. There's a practical reason for this. By puberty—reached around the age eight or nine—almost half of a group's males will be old enough to venture off to start a new life outside their home or "natal" group, either by pairing up with a female acquaintance from another group, or as a sole male on the lookout for a new group.

Females will make a "transfer" to another group, preferably led by a competent silverback, who will welcome her in. Alternatively, a female might transfer to a new group with a sole male. In order for emigrating gorillas to start a new life in this way, they will have had to master basic survival skills—chief among these being parenting, group collaboration, and foraging.

Experiences in the formative years determine whether they become leaders, followers, loners or family

Some males never settle down and wander as "lone males." Others may experiences a period of solitude but, eventually, take up a partnership with an emigrating female in a similar situation, or join an all-male group.

The course of a gorilla's life is fairly well set by adolescence. Experiences in the formative years determine whether they become leaders, followers, loners, or family types. Could insufficient playface practice as an infant later cost a lone male when courting? Could poor grooming skills come back to haunt the female who never gets the silverback? Maybe.

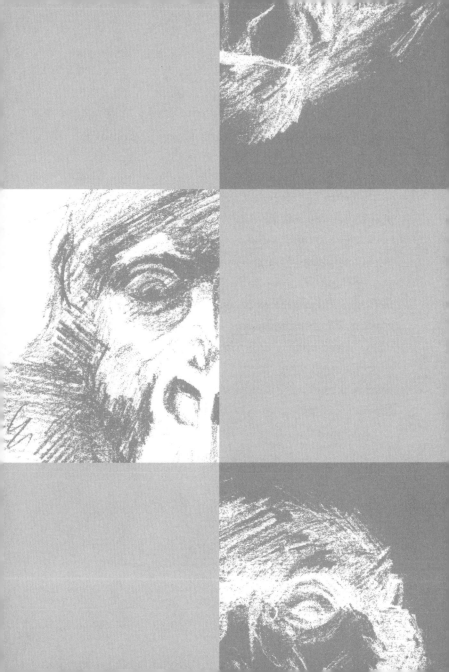

chapter two

family ties

Remember the feeling of dread upon hearing your father's heavy footfalls dead-silencing a midnight pillow fight? The door flies open. Lights flash. Big Trouble.

Now, imagine that you're a cheeky young gorilla who has just roused your silverback father from his cherished midday nap, just because you were bored.

Really Big Trouble?   Not exactly.

Gorillas are powerfully calm parents. They don't tend to lose their cool and show remarkable patience. Gorillas don't hit their young. As parents, they can be mistaken for a set of monkey bars, trampolines, bulls-eye targets, a pacifier, a tug-of-war rope, or even a napkin. Gorilla parents will not strike back. Instead, they use the "Gentle Rebuff": an almost Zen-like non-response to the nerve-jangling provocations of the young being... well, young.

Virtually every whining moment of a gorilla infant's first two months is spent either cradled in his mother's arms or clutched under her chest. They're 24/7 strapped-on, hand-clenched-on belly-hair, close to their moms. The result is "secure attachment," the magic ingredient that fosters confidence and adaptability to change. Sure, there's discipline, but discipline in the form of a hard stare or maybe a serious grunt. Dian Fossey observed that mountain gorillas nurture confidence by striking a "balance of discipline and affection." In this chapter on parenting we will explore how gorillas strike that balance— to great success.

the gentle rebuff

As long as kids test boundaries, they will test parents' nerves. Tantrums ensue, followed by admonishment, ending with commiseration. In this regard, the young gorilla seems to be just as pesky and persistent as his little human cousins. Dian Fossey observed that this parent-child tug-of-

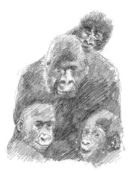

war spiked in the middle to the end of the infant's second year, when mothers are less responsive to demands but still provide necessities such as milk, warmth, grooming, rest, and protection.

Gorillas don't sweat the small stuff. Superfluous requests get a gentle rebuff (similar to their human counterparts who might ignore the whimpering of a dawdling child), or the gentle brushing away of an infant clamoring for milk.

To illustrate, a typical scenario might be a mother going about her business—feeding, resting, looking after the silverback's emotional needs. She encounters the histrionics of a screaming youngster demanding attention or milk or play. She simply ignores the infant as if she had just pushed the mute button—she stays strong and carries on. She knows the infant has no genuine need, so she will not respond with

The other night I ate at a real nice family restaurant.
Every table had an argument going.
—George Carlin

genuine concern—anger or otherwise. The infant desists…
much of the time. But if the infant persists, there's always the
tried-and-true pig grunt that communicates annoyance.

In a study by Alison Fletcher (of University College
Chester, England) on mountain gorilla mother-infant
relationships, infant tantrums involved "screaming, rolling
on the ground, pulling and shaking nearby vegetation."
(Note here that primatologists refer to young gorillas up
to about three years of age as infants.) When annoyed,
gorilla mothers will start with a pig grunt—a series of short,
rough guttural grunts—which may get amped up if the
infant doesn't respond. The most extreme consequence for
bad behavior might be a threat bite; a brisk movement of a
mother's head toward the infant, with open mouth, which is
more of a squeeze than a bite and doesn't hurt the infant….
This behavior might be likened to a human parent taking her
child firmly by the arm and saying "Now, that's enough!"

In the decades observing gorillas in captivity, I only

once witnessed a silverback striking a young gorilla—in this case a juvenile that was harassing a five-month-old female. In captivity, gorillas have been known to quarrel and attack for no obvious reason. I remember one such horrific incident, at the San Diego Zoo—an awfully aggressive display between a silverback and a female we had recently introduced into his enclosure. He was so rough with her, actually pushing her in the ground, that zoo workers resorted to splashing him with water to protect her. Again, that was behavior of gorillas in captivity, and likely products of emotional or psychological distress.

Most remarkably, mountain gorillas (in the wild) have never been documented hitting their young. In the 22 months she spent watching mountain gorilla mothers and infants, Alison Fletcher never once saw a mother strike or bite her young offspring. She also found that whining and tantrum–throwing infants got no more milk than those who were less demanding. The number of maternal rebuffs or amount of infant whimpering had no significant effect, in the end, on how much suckling the infant ultimately received. Mothers very rarely pig-grunted a "No" in response to an infant's request for suckling in the first year, but prevented or stopped infants suckling during years two and three. A few mothers never pig-grunted during the entire infancy age. Inevitably, though, the mother wins. After age two, most infants started rescheduling attempts for milk when it best suited the mother.

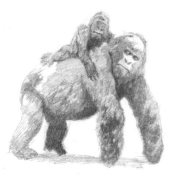

thisclose

Gorilla mothers are obsessed with keeping close to their young. But with relatively few real dangers threatening their offspring, why would they feel a need for constant proximity? Primatologists chalk it up as a selected behavior needed to develop survival skills crucial to thriving in gorilla groups and beyond. Being secure and mollycoddled as an infant, the theory goes, builds the confidence to deal with the rigors of life. Without it—as in the case of orphaned gorilla infants, for example—things can get grim. Dian Fossey wrote, for example, about a 38-month orphan who had changed from a "happy, outgoing social youngster into a pathetically withdrawn and sickly infant."

When she is one month old, an infant's hands are far too weak to grasp her mother's hair, so mothers constantly carry or cradle the newborn. And when she's untethered, she sets her infant down, no more than a few feet away, and only for short periods. As the months pass, the mother gorilla slowly extends the invisible leash, inch by inch. It's as if there's a built-in alarm that goes off when the infant wanders. Fletcher, who specializes in gorilla social development, found that mountain gorilla mothers keep infants younger than five months old within five feet, then, by eight months, they are permitted a wandering range of approximately 20 feet. Fletcher suggested that this close proximity ensures that the infant gets fed, but also learns the basics of eating plants and socializing through the mother's example.

She also found that mothers do a lot of rolling on the ground, playing horse, playing with infants' hands and feet and tickling in the first five months of the young gorilla's life. By age one, infants get into more physical play with their mothers, like jumping on the mother's big, trampoline-like belly. By two years, most infants dive into play with their peers, and play with their mothers tapers off significantly.

Gorillas may have the answer to the age-old question: Are little girls easier than little boys? For reasons that aren't clear, male gorilla infants tend to be mama's boys. One study found that gorilla mothers tend to invest more time and energy in male infants than in females. Males are carried under the chest longer than females. Mothers spend more time in contact with boys than with girls, and groom them more than they do their girls. But they also let male infants stray further than they let female infants. Mothers tend to restrain males more than they do females, perhaps because male infants play more often with older gorillas.

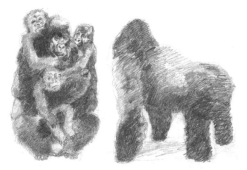

NURTURING NEURONS...

Some brain research backs up the developmental importance of secure attachment in early childhood. Allan Schore, a psychiatrist at the University of California at Los Angeles School of Medicine, suggests that secure nurturing can affect the formation of the brain's neural pathways in children up to two years old in ways that help them cope with stresses, as well as good and bad changes, all key to a child's ability to learn. This is no surprise to Alice Honig, a professor of child psychology at the University of Syracuse and author of *Secure Relationships: Nurturing Infant-Toddler Attachment in Early Care Settings*. "Successful secure attachments are at the core of bringing up well-adjusted and confident kids," she said in an interview.

socially groomed

It seems that preening is not just about looking good—at least for gorillas. Preening has strong social underpinnings as well. In contrast to human hugging, kissing, or putting hair in pigtails, gorilla parental grooming (probing, stroking, and cuddling) is a common form of motherly contact. Grooming the youngest entails: inspecting the bottom, genital areas, and hairy parts of the head, legs, and arms to tease out debris such as plant parts, dirt, and parasitic insects. This habit becomes socialized despite the fact that as infants get older, the parental grooming tails off, and juveniles persist to groom one another.

the invisible teacher

Gorilla parents seem to be the opposite of pushy. They let their young figure it out on their own—from finding the rights foods or playmates or making a nest for napping.

Dario Maestripieri of the University of Chicago found that in all major areas of social behavior—feeding, playing, napping, foraging, and communicating—infants take the initiative. He looked at two-to-four-year-old western lowland gorillas interacting with mothers and found that mothers control an infant's social interaction only during rough play, or when the infant is near an unrelated dominant male gorilla. In almost all other cases, the infant, not the mother, initiates social behaviors. Mothers never clearly encourage, or discourage, their offspring's behavior in food-sharing, facial expressions, play, or spending time with others. They intervene, but only when the young are in danger.

Maestripieri and others have noted that this non-interference opens up opportunities for exploration, which encourages self-teaching—a kind of teaching without teaching called "scaffolding." In the entire year that George

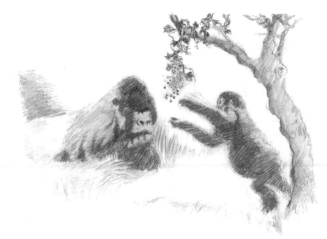

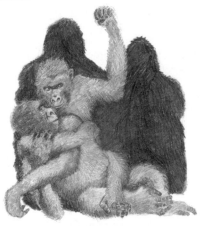

Schaller lived among mountain gorillas, he rarely saw mothers get involved in an infant's foraging. When he did, it was so remarkable that he made special note of it, as when a five-month-old struggled to uproot a stem and his mother eventually snapped it off for him, or when a mother snatched a leaf petiole from an infant (this part of the plant is typically ignored by adults).

dad, the psychological buffer

Some of the most violent fights ever observed among gorillas have been over an infant threatened by an outsider male or human. The silverback lives a fairly docile life, guiding the group to feeding spots, sleeping spots, and sunning spots. But he's also the power broker when fights break out, especially when the young are involved.

Silverbacks become what Kelly Stewart of the University of California, Davis, calls a "psychological buffer" or an "attachment figure" for the infant as the mother weans the child. Stewart, who studies how silverbacks and youngsters relate, found that silverbacks are key to cooling down squabbling youngsters through what's called "control intervention," which can involve subtle cues: a stare, a grunt, or a movement toward the two quarrelers.

If the fight is over a contested object—such as food—most control interventions will result in the younger gorilla keeping the object. Stewart found that about half of all control interventions are done by the silverback. By the age of three, the time spent in close proximity and in contact with the mother drops off, and the amount of time with the silverback increases.

sleeping arrangements

For some (human) adults, getting kids to sleep alone at night is fraught with worry, guilt, and frustration. Start newborns in a crib right from day one? Share the parents' bed? But for

43

how long?...12 days, 12 months, 12 years?

Gorillas sleep with their young past the age it would seem necessary. Typically, infant gorillas sleep in their mothers' nests until they are two to three years old—in human years, around seven or eight. But gorilla infants practice building their own nests as early as eight months old. Two-year–olds build nests close to—sometimes connected to—their mothers' but usually hop into the mothers' nest, built knowingly bigger to accommodate the two.

Eventually, the young will build their own nests, separate from, but in very close proximity to their mothers. Juveniles (young gorillas over the age of three) still occasionally sleep with their mothers, especially if the mother doesn't have an infant.

custom-made bedding

Gorillas build fresh nests every time they sleep—typically for a midday rest, then at dusk. Ground nests are made by bending foliage in toward the center of an oval shape and matting it down, creating a mounded rim.

Tree nests, more commonly used by lighter members of

the group and groups without a male (presumably because it may provide more safety from predators), are made by bending branches in a fabric–like form to create a springy mattress.

GROUND NEST

1 Bend foliage in toward center to form oval shape.

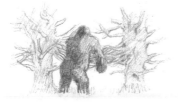

2 Matt down, creating molded rim.

TREE NEST

1 Bend surrounding branches and inter-twine to form fabric-like mattress.

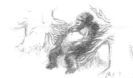

2 Continue to add branches to support weight of nester.

gorilla and human parenting

Dr. Alice Sterling Honig, professor emerita of child development at Syracuse University, was asked to offer some advice on how parents can form secure attachments with their young children. The table below draws comparisons between Honig's approaches and those observed by wild gorillas.

INFANTS

	GORILLA	**HUMAN**
HOLDING	Carry your infant in the ventral position or cradle him for the first year non-stop. Let him hang on you, climb on you, bounce on your belly. Keep him within a few feet of you, as you are the most important role model.	Cuddle your baby. Lift baby onto your shoulder so she nuzzles your neck. Carry her in a kangaroo pouch against your chest while working at chores. When sitting in a rocking chair, drape her over your belly. Hold her on your hip while walking about.
NURSING	Let the infant suckle any time he wants, even if you're hungry, cold, and tired. After the first year, ignore unnecessary requests, but nurse at intervals that are necessary.	Nurse baby in tune with her unique tempo. Some babies are "snackers." They suck briefly, then turn to look about. Others gulp intensely and for a long period. Notice and get comfortable with your baby's tempo.
TOUCHING	Tickle feet and hands in a playful manner. Groom head, neck, limbs, and bottom regularly to remove insects and debris, as well as to introduce him to the social importance of grooming later on in life.	Massage each baby limb using nonallergenic oils. Massage eases colic pains and body tensions. Use long palm strokes on back, belly, arms, and legs. Talk to your baby lovingly as you massage.

YOUNG KIDS

PLAYING

GORILLA

Peek–a–boo, king-of-the-mountain. Do not discourage infant from tossing vegetation to get your attention or the attention of other group members. Allow infant to pick food scraps off your lap and, later, to try out his first attempts at picking out the most nutritious parts of plants. Let him make mistakes. He'll learn through watching others and trial and error.

HUMAN

Play partnership games such as peek-a-boo; pat-a-cake; this little piggy goes to market. Arrange cooking games. Enlist your child as a "helper" to shred lettuce or make hamburger patties. Help your child feel secure in the bosom of important family activities.

GROWING INDEPENDENCE

After the first year, slowly permit your infant to explore his environment and to interact with others. He should learn on his own, at his own pace. Do not intrude on his playing (e.g., swinging on branches, walking on fallen tree trunks, flinging foliage) unless he is in danger.

Encourage more mature behaviors by tiny steps. If you are intrusive in demanding instant correct handling of a toy, such as a ring stack, the child becomes discouraged and feels untrusted. Your patience, kindness, and nurturing will guarantee secure attachment to you, letting your child grow up as a kind, caring human being, able to give and receive love.

PROTECTION

If an infant gets hurt, swoop him up, remove him, and caress. If he is harmed or threatened by others, intercede immediately, and wait for the silver-back to either use control intervention or, in most dire cases, full-on assault.

Empathize with your child's feelings. Do not call children "sissy"; do not ridicule a child's fears. Be calm. Be reassuring. Stroke your child's hair to soothe scared or hurting feelings. Children with empathetic mothers are much more pro-social and positive with peers years later.

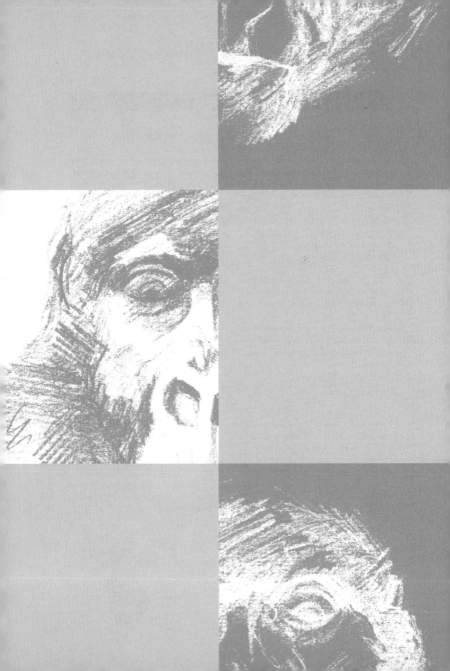

the silverback

All leaders—human and gorilla—seem to perform a perpetual balancing act. They need to simultaneously maintain a certain friendliness and earn loyalty and trust among their followers, without losing the ability to wield power (even with friends). They need to ensure the group stays intact, cooperative, on course.

The silverback's job as peacekeeper is to manage all members in the hierarchical line, keep them safe and well fed and, most important, put a quick end to any squabbling, which could weaken and distract the group. The social hierarchy of gorilla groups goes roughly like this, from top to bottom: silverback, blackback, adult female with infant, adult female without offspring, juveniles, and infants.

Martha Robbins, of the Max Planck Institute for Evolutionary Anthropology, suggests that well-defined

You can't be a leader unless there are people who are willing to be followers. Followers let someone else be a leader and give up their desires and abilities to lead."
—Karen Izod, consultant, executive coaching,
The Tavistock Institute, London

dominance and rank levels are what make gorilla groups stable. This does not mean that silverbacks are bullies. Despite holding the top spots, male gorillas use physical aggression against other males as a last resort only; for example, when competing for a mate. Typically, males "coexist through avoidance or tolerance of one another rather than by using frequent, active antagonism or by forming strong supportive groups," Robbins writes.

When silverbacks speak, others listen. Their sounds range from deafening roars to barely audible grunts. In pioneering work, Dian Fossey categorized 16 distinct vocalizations. She found that silverbacks do most of the vocalizing and were also most likely to elicit a response to their vocalizations. Further studies, including those by Alexander Harcourt and Kelly Stewart, found that all group members responded more to silverback calls than to calls of lower-ranked group members. Mothers, however, nearly always respond to vocalizations by their young infants.

One may speculate that this is a product of subservience to the silverback—or, worse, a knee-jerk habit borne of fear. But considering how seldom silverbacks exert physical force on their group members, it is likely a behavior that suggests well-oiled social cohesion among gorilla groups that require one indisputable leader.

"A good leader will bring enemies and friends together, then push them away again. Leaders can break up normally antagonistic relationships."
—Ron Riggio

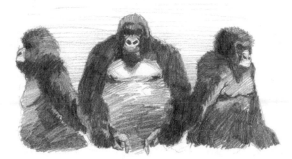

LEADER MOTIVE PROFILE

The *Leader Motive Profile* (LMP), described by David McClelland in the 1970s, holds that a combination of motives make a good predictor of a successful leader. The chart below describes some apparent LMPs for humans and gorillas.

gorilla	human
GAINING POWER	
Motivated by being the most influential to gain power, especially among females	Highly motivated by status and influence over people
SPREADING POWER	
Motivated by having as many off-spring as possible, and pro-tecting them	Believes that power should not be abused
HOLDING POWER	
Motivated to defend weaker group members for the good of the group	More highly motivated to attain power than to form close ties with followers

Maintaining harmony in the group means protecting mates, offspring, and status. For example, silverbacks break up female–female conflicts so frequently and so effectively, through what's known as "control interventions," that conflicts more often end with no real winner or loser (see sidebar opposite). For the most part, silverbacks do this by not favoring one female over another, sometimes punishing both the aggressor and victim, and almost always showing support for the younger of the two squabblers. This effectively reduces the benefits of female coalitions, protects the underdogs, and discourages bullying.

David Watts, of Yale University, found that 84 percent of all silverback interventions involved breaking up fights between females, and that males used control interventions about 75 percent of the time, supporting neither female. Predictably, they were more successful at resolving conflicts when they got physically involved—approaching, displaying, or even grabbing or hitting females—than when they merely vocalized. Males also broke up squabbles more than three times more often with conflicts involving large female coalitions than with small coalitions. When males intervened in fights between immatures, they most often supported the younger of the two, regardless of who was the aggressor.

chest-beating: the art of the bluff

Silverbacks produce chest beats that resonate like drums, amplified by air sacs inflated in the throat. The chest beats can be heard from a mile away.

Chest beating is not necessarily a warm-up to battle. It can, at times, be a bluff used to avoid an escalation or a confrontation, or simply a loud way of making one's presence clearly known. It might be used, for instance, when spotting a suspected predator or encountering a lone outsider male. George Schaller suggests that these displays are a way to let off steam when agitated or when frustratingly stuck between the conflicting desires of "fight and flight." While fierce and threatening in countenance, most displays are relatively benign (although occasionally a member is injured in the running part of the display due to the close proximity of other members) and don't result in mortal combat.

There seems to be something contagious in chest-beating, and it can be practiced as a ritualized group behavior borne of fear and alarm. Silverbacks are known for the most powerful and full display, but juveniles, females and even infants have been seen carrying out parts of the display. Outsiders from different groups have been observed taking part, as well.

Schaller broke the chest-beating display down into nine steps, although he only observed silverbacks completing the entire sequence. More often, partial displays—involving just a few of these steps—are carried out. Displays by females are shorter, rarer, and less intense than displays by males.

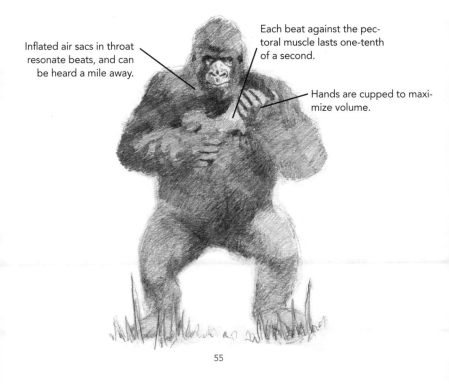

Inflated air sacs in throat resonate beats, and can be heard a mile away.

Each beat against the pectoral muscle lasts one-tenth of a second.

Hands are cupped to maximize volume.

SCHALLER'S 9-STEP CHEST-BEATING DISPLAY*

Below is the sequence of nine steps silverbacks take when threatened. The center piece, and most spectacular step is the actual chest-beating. Juveniles and other group members often engage in a partial display.

—*Adapted from *The Mountain Gorilla: Ecology and Behavior*, George Schaller

1 Hooting: Soft "hoots" through pursed lips can begin the display, and can quicken. Could be a tip-off to other group members to a threat.

2 "Symbolic feeding": Hooting halts, and gorilla places a piece of vegetation, or even non-food item, in the mouth, and pretends to eat. Only done in about 10% of full displays. Classic "displacement activity."

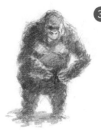

3 Rising: Rises on hind legs and stands, with head and torso leaning forward, right before climax of display.

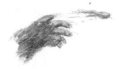

4 Throwing: Tosses a piece of vegetation, up to 20 feet, or simply flicks it. May also simulate throwing motion with nothing in hand.

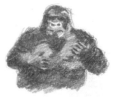

5 Chest beating: Fast hitting or slapping on chest with both hands cupped, just below the pectoral chest muscles. May beat sitting or standing, and may also beat with just one hand. Hands are beat from about six inches of the chest and are struck one after the other. Schaller described the sound as a "hollow pok-pok-pok." Typically about eight slaps long.

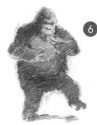

6 Leg kicking: Kicks one leg in the air while chest-beating.

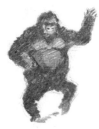

7 Running: Lateral running, during or just after chest beating.

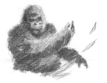

8 Slapping and tearing: Slapping or tearing at nearby vegetation with a forceful swipe while running.

9 Ground thumping: Ends the display by striking one blow to the ground with the palm.

Silverbacks use other intimidation tactics, as well. "Bluff charges" involve charging up to 80 feet toward a target without making contact. The long, hard stare is a threat, too; the longer it lasts, the greater the intended threat.

outside competition

Mountain gorilla silverbacks are fairly good about sharing territory with other groups, typically avoiding conflict by moving along without incident when encountering another group.

Because of a hospitable environment, gorillas don't need to resort to random violence to antagonize competitors. They coexist with other animals in relative peace.

They are more likely to hold their ground, and fight when protecting an infant or a threatened female than they would on other common encounters such as territorial disputes over prime foraging spots. I witnessed this first-hand. During a visit to Republic of Congo, I observed a silverback and a three-year-old male. They were glued to

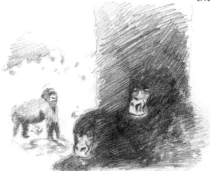

each other. When I approached them, only slightly, the male charged me. I dropped my camera and fell to my knees. He halted about eight feet from me, then turned around to join the young male. That was his way of holding his ground, yet not inflicting harm on an intruder.

Pascale Sicotte, who studied gorilla group encounters in Rwanda and Zaire, found that 74 percent of all encounters involve threatening displays like as strutting, hooting, and chest beating. Seventeen percent involve physical forms of aggression, like as slapping. Aggressive encounters seem be driven by males preventing their "available" females from transferring to another group, or a group attempting to lure a female to transfer into its group.

Interestingly, the higher the number of females without dependent offspring in one or both groups, the greater the incidence of aggressive behavior between males of the groups. Groups with fewer potential female migrants tend to have less fractious encounters with other groups.

According to Joan Silk, a professor of anthropology at the University of California, Los Angeles, random attacks—for many animals contesting limited resources (such as food)—are an efficient way for aggressors to wreak the greatest amount of havoc for their victims and exert their dominance with fairly little effort. Gorillas, who have relatively little competition for food and few predators, due to their hospitable environment (and, possibly, by their natures), experience little in the way of random aggression.

charisma and presence

Silverbacks are the magnet of a group, attracting infants to the oldest females. He's the one most followed and most listened to. Just as charismatic people seem to take up more space than followers, silverbacks have ways of creating this aura as well. Conspicuous examples include making lots of noise and commotion (chest-beating or water splashing).

Another display of his dominance is his "strut"—a rigid walk, with arms bent outwards, to make the arms appear bigger. The strut is performed in different contexts—before copulation, during play, in the presence of humans, or as a signal to the group that it's time to get up and move on. Schaller suggests that the strut makes a gorilla look more powerful and is also a way of showing off.

. . . . . .

THE SILVERBACKS AMONG US

Look confident, not cocky. Look assertive, not aggressive. Look like "I belong here, this is my territory." It's more about a confident walk, not a swagger.

—Marjorie Brady, executive coach

Leaders are often people who somehow assume a bigger presence, who appear to take up greater floor space. People who cease to be leaders appear smaller, and have a smaller physical presence."

—Karen Izod, consultant, executive coaching, The Tavistock Institute, London

With the silverback gone, group members are effectively orphaned, splitting off to join other groups, to brave it alone, or to form another group.

Silverbacks use special positioning to demand attention. They often rise from eating or resting and stand stiff-legged. Then they wait. This prompts others to follow within minutes. If the silverback gets up abruptly, group members will follow more quickly. When the group is moving briskly, the silverback typically leads. When the group lolls about, the silverback brings up the rear or is in the middle.

sans silverback: the power vacuum

What happens when the patriarch falls?

Without the silverback, subordinate members become effectively orphaned, splitting off and joining other groups as low-ranking individuals. Infants of females emigrating to a new group are vulnerable to infanticide by that group's reigning silverback, (this is particularly true among mountain gorillas). In general, females don't stay together for life but opt instead to go off on their own to seek out a new group or a solitary male. Even groups losing a lead silverback (for example due to a fatal fall or infection) left behind with only

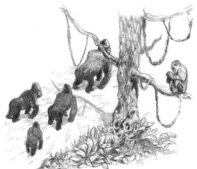

a sole surviving silverback, see defections and can ultimately become weakened and vulnerable to aggression from other groups. In other cases, a dissolution of a group leads to non-silverback males forging out from the group to form their own groups or face a life as lone, unattached males.

There are exceptions, of course. Juichi Yamigawa observed one group of eastern lowland gorillas whose silverback died. The remaining group members, just females and juveniles, lived alone for 29 months, despite persistent efforts by neighboring males to take over the group. These females and their young had been driven to sleep in trees, but resumed sleeping in ground nests when a new silverback finally joined the group successfully and became their leader.

"If you can't work with different factions, you're toppled."
—Ron Riggio

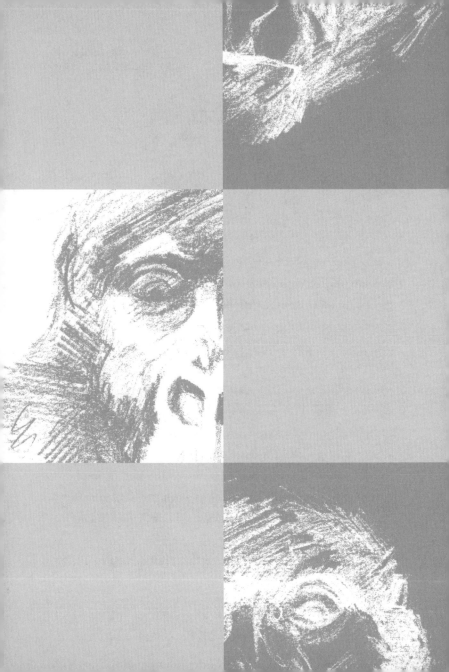

chapter four

eating out

What does a 400-pound, tooth-flashing gorilla—built to maul anything at will—hunt down for his next meal? Nothing that will bite him back. It's mostly just leaves, stems, roots, and fruit. Gorillas are vegans.

A wealth of field research exists on surveying and tracking the diet of gorillas—and on the sophisticated and dexterous preparation of their foods. What the research adds up to is that gorillas are very sophisticated and accomplished foragers.

From hundreds of plants, gorillas find the right balance of low fat, high fiber, and high protein. To achieve this, they have turned food prep into a high art, with an estimated 78 separate hand-processing maneuvers to extract the right stuff from the useless stuff. They even make leaf sandwiches.

And consider this humbling estimate: the average wild gorilla's diet follows dietary guidelines of the U.S. National Research Council of Health more closely than that of an estimated 97 percent of Americans. As concern surrounding the obesity epidemic mounts, public health initiatives are promoting diets of lower-fat, higher-fiber and, naturally, all-vegetable protein—diets, incidentally, which are quite similar to what gorillas have been eating all along.

So, what if we were to follow the gorillas' foraging trail and venture further into the forest? Imagine... poached thistle, roasted wild celery on a bed of bamboo shoots, iron-enriched clay mousse. Not exactly molecular gastronomy, but through a clearing in the dense thicket of research on gorilla foraging, one can easily imagine bamboo shoots becoming the next arugula.

That may sound like a tempting idea, but it's implausible. Our gullets and digestive tracts cannot tolerate so much fiber. The other inconvenience of following a typical gorilla diet is that most gorilla plant foods, even some wild fruits, taste bitter or sour to the human palate. Thousands of years of cultivating fruits and vegetables—increasing crop yields and, in many foods, sugar content—

have removed some tastes of the wild from our plates. The ultimate barrier to eating all that gorillas eat is that some gorilla plant foods are toxic to humans.

. . . . . .

PLANT FOODS AND PREVENTING CANCER

"There is convincing evidence that diets high in vegetables and/or fruits protect against cancers of the mouth and pharynx, oesophagus, lung, stomach and colon and rectum (in particular, the evidence is strongest for raw vegetables, green vegetables, allium vegetables [the onion family], carrots, tomatoes and citrus fruit). Such diets probably also protect cancers of the larynx, pancreas, breast and bladder, and possibly against cancers of the liver, ovary, endometrium, cervix, prostrate, thyroid, and kidney."

—From *Food, Nutrition and the Prevention of Cancer: A Global Perspective*, published by World Cancer Research Fund

what gorillas eat

For over four decades, primatologists have traipsed long hours in cold, soggy African rain forests with an archeologist's zeal to catalogue what gorillas eat. Extracting each new piece of the dietary puzzle must have been as painstaking as teasing out ceramic shards from bone dry earth and, surely, has involved a lot of waiting, tracking, and poking.

Over the years, gorilla plant-food diet lists have grown, with newer, longer, and more complete lists supplanting old ones. It's been a meticulous hunt for every newly identifiable fruit, seed, leaf, shoot, fern, pith, stem, twig, fungus, bark, palm, thistle, trunk, nettle, and root and—even dirt—that gorillas pop into their mouths.

Diets of gorilla subspecies differ according to their habitats and abilities. In general, lowland gorillas tend to eat much more fruit than mountain gorillas (who tend to stick to foliage and stem foods), mainly because fruits are more plentiful in their habitats. Some gorillas, particularly western lowland gorillas, have even been spotted eating ants and termites. Mountain gorilla favorites include bamboo shoots (an excellent source of protein), wild celery, thistles, shelf fungus, nettles, and blackberries.

Like us, individual gorillas have different tastes and diets. But unlike us, they consume a far wider variety of plant foods. Elizabeth Williamson of the University of Stirling (UK) collected data over six years in Gabon. She found that 98 percent of dung samples of western lowland gorillas contained fruit seeds. Of the 182 plant foods they eat, 95 are *different* fruits, stretching the apple-a-day maxim to quite an extreme. Yale anthropologist David Watts, after logging in 2,400 hours watching three mountain gorilla groups eat in Rwanda, found that one group ate foods from 38 distinct plant species while another group ate foods from 24.

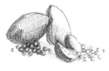

In general, lowland gorillas tend to eat much more fruit than mountain gorillas, mainly because the fruits are rich in some of their habitats.

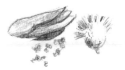

Some mountain gorilla favorites: wild blackberry, wild celery, and thistle.

Some gorillas, particularly western lowland gorillas, have even been spotted eating ants and termites.

FALLBACK FOODS

According to foraging theory, when preferred foods are unavailable, and when excessive energy is needed to find these foods, simian foragers adapt by searching for more readily available, yet second-rate, foods. Juichi Yamagiwa, of Kyoto University, found that when fruit supplies are short for the eastern lowland gorillas in Zaire's tropical rain forests, they rely on "fallback foods" and a more diverse diet including a greater number of species of leaves, bark—and even ants, termites, and other insects. Likewise, mountain gorillas gorge on young bamboo shoots, which make up 90 percent of their diet when they're in season. But when the shoots are gone, they resort to other foods.

In a nutshell, the gorilla diet is low in fat, high in fiber and protein. David Popovich and David Jenkins, of the University of Toronto, estimated that fiber makes up more than half of the core diet of the western lowland gorilla; protein about 35 percent; and fat, just over 2.5 percent.

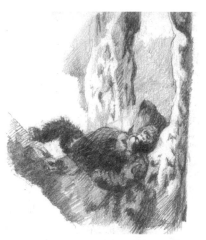

Health organizations recommend that the human diet should ideally comprise about 15 percent of dietary fiber, with 10–35 percent of calories from protein, 20–30 percent from fat and 45–65 percent from carbohydrates. While gorillas have rarely been spotted drinking water from a pool,

"Gorillas are a part of their ecologies. We fight ours. ...
A lot of going forward means going back."
—David Jenkins, University of Toronto

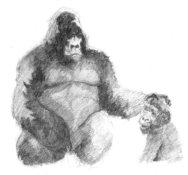

they get copious amounts from plants. British primatologist Alan Goodall estimated that adult male mountain gorillas eat about 30 kilograms of food a day, from which up to 27 liters is water.

Gorillas can be tempted into eating fast food, just like us. As impressive as their diets are in the wild, gorillas take on our vices when in captivity, and can easily be seduced by the same foods that we like—meat, eggs, even popcorn. Predictably, many gorillas in captivity are heavier and have more chronic diseases than their wild cousins. Zoos have taken great strides to introduce a more native diet in order to help prevent nutrition-related illnesses.

SMALL PHARMA

"Eating so much fiber can't be easy on the stomach. It seems that gorillas have found a clever antidote, though. William Mahaney, of York University (Ontario, Canada), found that mountain gorillas lick up a clay rich in iron and containing aluminum and magnesium—making for a chemical composition similar to the antacid medication Kaopectate. The clay is believed to adsorb toxins. It is also believed to help manage dehydration during drier months which is when, perhaps not coincidentally, it is typically ingested.

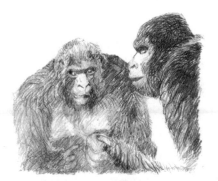

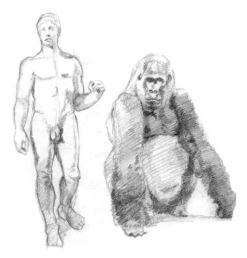

MEASURING UP

homo sapiens   wild gorilla

Average weight (adult male)
180 lb   337 lb

Average life expectancy
74 years (male, U.S.)   27 years

Average daily red meat, poultry and fish intake
8.8 ounces*   0.0 ounces

Average fat intake (as % of total calories)
33.4%   2.0%*
*Economic Research Service, U.S. Dept. of Agriculture, 2005

foraging: the art of the hunt

Foraging dictates the daily routine of gorillas, influencing how far they travel, where they sun, and with whom they rest. This aspect of gorilla life is so important, that becoming a silverback requires being a discerning and successful forager in addition to being a leader, a protector, and siring new group members.

Foraging usually entails settling into an area of favorite plants, gathering the right parts—and usually leaving a mess of broken foliage behind. Sometimes lighter group members (this is especially true of the lowland gorillas) eat in trees up to 40 meters tall. After the meal, they're off again, led by the silverback, in pursuit of a new eating spot. As they trek through the different landscapes of their range, which vary from steep mountain slopes to river valleys, meadows, and bamboo groves, gorillas take part in a lifelong field trip identifying plants and plant parts and learning how to prep them.

A study of the diets of western lowland gorillas found that of the 182 plant foods they eat, 95 are different fruits.

SMART SHOPPERS

American ecologist Amy Vedder spent an entire year in Africa's Virunga Mountains watching what mountain gorillas ate and collecting samples of plants left behind in their nests. She also followed the gorillas or their trails for 311 days and discovered a link between what the gorillas ate and how they foraged for food. She found that these gorillas spent more time in areas containing high-protein and diverse foods, and that their ranging patterns were created based on the locales of the most preferred foods. They spent almost 80 percent of their time foraging five types of plant foods that, hardly a coincidence, also happened to contain the highest protein concentrations of the 30 most common plants in their diet.

* * * * * *

Gorillas forage in home ranges, which vary depending on the group size and the silverback leader's foraging style.

Mountain gorillas' home ranges, for instance, average around 10 square miles, and they visit areas with the highest quality or greatest diversity of foods. Daily treks range from barely moving (100 yards) to up to three miles.

Although they appear to make arabesque loops through ranges, their movements are hardly a random wild-goose chase. In these twists and turns are recognizable patterns. After a group feeds on (and pretty much trashes) an area, it can revisit that patch weeks or months later when the vegetation is recovered and grown—in some cases even more fully foliated—thus primed for another round of feeding. It works out well for the hunters and hunted.

Gorillas, in this way, could be the world's first sustainable-agriculture developers.

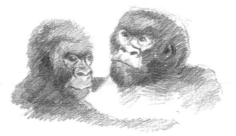

the art of food prepping

It's humbling to see how more advanced gorillas are than humans in their food-prepping skills. Teasing pith from stems and extracting the youngest and most nutritious leaves, for example, are multiple-step skills—learned, honed, and improvised. These skills add up to an impressive repertoire of culinary handiwork, shared among group members and passed on to the next generation. Indeed, a young gorilla first samples solid foods by picking scraps off his mother's lap.

What struck me about the mountain gorillas I observed in the wild was how enormously destructive they were to the plant life as they entered (or, rather, trampled into) feeding areas, given their great size and that much of the plants they ate were at ground level. At times, I wondered whether this was done to stake their territory within a rich feeding area, or if it were simply a product of their girth and weight. In any case, though, once they got settled in at their respective "seats," their plundering of the plant-life would give way to a most impressive opposing display of delicate—and even fastidious—handiwork in the preparing of their food.

What's particularly impressive is how quickly wild mountain gorillas recognize the most preferred parts of edible

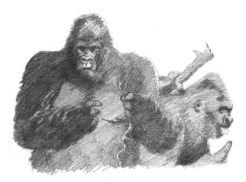

plants and the efficiency, precision, and great dexterity with which they prepare their food. It's quite amazing to watch these enormous creatures mastering such fine hand and arm motor skills—and keen eyesight and muscle memory—that are not dissimilar, really, to that of fine embroidery or even the tying of trout flies.

What I observed, clearly, were skills accrued and finely tuned over years. And it was not only self-learned. The young were alert students as their mature handlers demonstrated foraging, prepping, and consumption. I was struck by a few three-year-olds glued to the silverbacks while eating. I assumed the young held on tightly simply because that's where the food was. And professional researchers have studied this as likely the case. But I cannot help think that the proximity must impart daily food preparation lessons for the young as well—lessons that have been passed on, quite likely, for thousands of generations.

Richard Byrne of the University of St Andrews (Scotland) spent more than 500 hours in Rwanda videotaping 44 mountain gorillas from infancy to adulthood. He identified 26 distinct leaf-processing actions and found that by combining these actions into different sequences, the mountain gorilla had developed 78 separate food-processing patterns. Byrne suggests that these complex skills helped the large, relatively slow gorilla survive as a species—by being able to manually pick out the nutritious plant parts from plants that have natural defenses (like needles, toxic plant parts, sheaths, and shells).

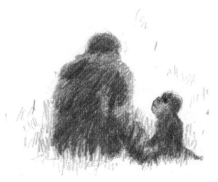

GORILLAS AND THE SLOW FOOD MOVEMENT

> "We are enslaved by speed and have all suc-
> cumbed to the same insidious virus: Fast
> Life, which disrupts our habits, pervades the
> privacy of our homes and forces us to eat Fast
> Foods. Our defense should begin at the table
> with Slow Food. Let us rediscover the flavors
> and savors of regional cooking and banish the
> degrading effects of Fast Food."
>
> —From the Slow Food International Manifesto

Finding the best food takes work. Many of the gorilla's favorite foods have prickly defenses that evolved against herbivores: tiny hooks, stings or needles, which require removal through a bit of manipulation to avoid smarting the mouth. They peel wild celery stalks, for example, and remove petioles (leaf stalks) from blackberries. They uproot certain plants, strip the roots, eat the high-protein insides, and discard the rest. Mountain gorillas have mastered the nutritious but tricky practice of consuming the stinging nettle (part of traditional diets in northern Europe for hundreds of years).

The mountain gorilla has at least 26 distinct leaf-
processing actions; combining these actions into
different sequences effectively disposes it to 78 separate
food-processing patterns.

how to eat a nettle without choking

During its life, a gorilla picks up an impressive repertoire
of plant-processing skills requiring delicate finger dexterity,
strong and firm arms, hands and fingers, and nimble lips
and teeth. According to psychologist Richard Byrne, of
the University of St Andrews (Scotland), the repertoire
of skills needed to do this starts early, and by age three
(equal to a seven-year-old child), they learn most of the key
handiwork techniques.

Byrne observed mountain gorillas taking these steps to
eat the leaves of the stinging nettle (Laportea alatipes). The
petiole is removed and the underside of the stinging leaf
is avoided.

HOW TO MAKE A NETTLE SANDWICH

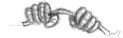

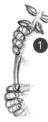

1 With one hand supporting the stem tightly at the roots, the other hand slides up along the stem, stripping off leaves.

2 The unwanted base of the leaves (the petioles) are held in one hand, with the preferred top ends sticking out, and then twisted off with the other hand. Unwanted base leaves are discarded.

3 The bundle of leaf tops is held loosely in one hand, and any debris is picked out with the other hand.

4 Leaves are pulled out of one hand with the other, and the bundle is formed into a sandwich—with stings cased by a single leaf, and non-stinging topside exposed. Bundled sandwich is popped into mouth.

aping a gorilla diet

For those who want to dive into high-vegetable, low-low-fat menus, an answer could lie in the so-called "portfolio diet,"*created by nutritionist David Jenkins and his team at the University of Toronto. The portfolio diet resembles the gorilla diet and has been found to promote health and lower the bad form of cholesterol.

Below is a sampling of foods subjects ate in David Jenkins' cholesterol-lowering portfolio diet studies. These foods are high in vegetable proteins, plant sterols, dietary fiber, antioxidants, folate and micro nutrients, and low in salt, sugars, saturated fats, trans fatty acids, and dietary cholesterol. A registered dietician could likely help create a complete meal plan based on these nutritional parameters.

The portfolio diet resembles the gorilla diet and has been found to promote health and lower the bad form of cholesterol.

A SIMULATED SIMIAN MENU

Breakfast: Hot oatbran cereal, soy beverage (such as soy milk), strawberries, psyllium, oat bran bread, plant- sterol-enriched margerine,** double-fruit jam, orange, Metamucil fiber supplement

Lunch: Sandwich made from soy deli slices, oat bran bread, lettuce, tomato, cucumber; soups include: lentil with curry, vegetable barley, minestrone with pasta, spicy black bean soup; soy hot dogs

Snacks: Almonds, soy beverage, fresh fruit

Dinner: Tofu bake with ratatouille (containing tofu, eggplant, onions and sweet peppers, pearled barley, vegetables, such as broccoli and cauliflower); ground tofu, vegetable curry, soy burger, northern beans, kidney beans; lentils, chickpeas, carrot, three-bean chili, okra, red pepper

* Menu included with permission of the author.
** Margerine used in this diet is enriched with plant sterols, found in leafy vetetables and vegetable oils.

I've witnessed captive gorillas consume human food—usually through unfortunate incidents when visitors at zoos would toss snacks into enclosures. As I learned just how varied the gorilla's natural diet is, I must admit I was tempted to create a diet that might be at once true to the staple of the gorilla's diet, yet palatable, digestible, and nutritious for people. Or, at least, to me.

So, I tried a modified version of the Jenkins diet. The best way to test this was to stick to such a diet religiously. The first few days started off well. I avoided my usual junk food and felt more alert. But I lost my religion after only about two weeks. Sadly, the diet never fully satisfied, and did not altogether agree with my gastro-intestinal system. Since that full-on gorilla diet, though, I do eat more nuts, whole grain, and legumes, and fruits. I also tend to eat four or five smaller meals during the day, instead of one or two very large ones. My diet is indeed closer to that of the gorilla's, and I believe I'm better off because of it.

Note, however, that there are a few things to consider when trying this diet. First, consult a registered nutritionist or physician—especially if you have a medical condition, such as high-cholesterol levels, or if you're pregnant. The

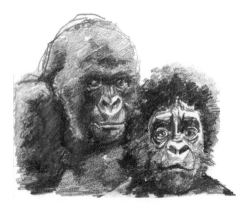

portfolio diet—which is about as close to the gorilla diet you can get with readily available foods—does not lower or raise HDL cholesterol, so people with low levels of this might look elsewhere to raise the HDL, like aerobic exercise and some cholesterol-reducing drugs. Additionally, Jenkins' diet calls for psyllium, a seed-grain fiber supplement, which may interact adversely with some drugs.

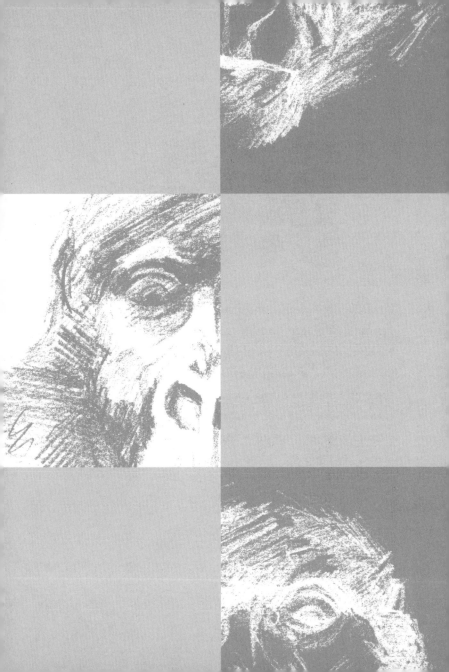

chapter five

beyond words

Words can mislead, misguide, misfire.

The good news is that only 7 percent of the information we receive from another person is verbal, according to UCLA psychologist Albert Mehrabian. So, considering that most of the information we send to others is nonverbal, why not look closely to those who've mastered a complex lexicon of body language?

Gorillas accurately and unambiguously send—and decode—hundreds of gestures and facial expressions and postures, and it's not all just chest beating and grunting. There are also subtler, and nuanced—though no less demonstrative—gestures, we might see a submissive bow of the head, a peacekeeping gesture, sticking out a tongue, a sign of amazement, and yawning, which might signify unease or stress.

ICONIC GESTURES: ORIGINS OF LANGUAGE?

A study by Joanne E. Tanner and Richard Byrne suggest that the iconic gestures (those representing action) of gorillas and other non-human primates may hold clues about the earliest forms of human communication.

These iconic gestures can be visual (stretching an arm in the direction you want someone to go) or tactile (pushing that someone in the intended direction). Among gorillas, tactile gestures were generally more effective, not surprisingly. Also, play-faces had a big role, often initiating an interaction. Combining a playface and at least one other gesture (such as a hug) led to greater subsequent contact than did the same gesture with no playface.

making faces

With some 30 highly innervated muscles, the human face is built to provide the widest range of expressiveness: from the Mona Lisa to The Scream. With relatively similar facial musculature, gorillas also rely on their face to express and communicate.

Looking to animals to learn about nonverbal communication is nothing new. Charles Darwin's pioneering work, *The Expressions of the Emotions in Man and Animals*, published in 1872, is a seminal work of early comparative psychology. In it, Darwin argued his foundational theory that basic facial expressions are universal, and that nonverbal forms of communication are species specific, not enculturated.

It's not surprising that gorillas share some of man's repertoire of facial expressions: smiles, laughter, anger, and uncertainty. For example, gorillas purse their lips against their teeth (called "lip-tucking"), when feeling uncertain. This is similar to "lip-compression," a human nonverbal indicator of uncertainty as well as grief, anger, or sadness. according to nonverbal communication expert David Givens' *The Nonverbal Dictionary*.

SLY SMILE

Monitoring and controlling of facial expressions begins between the ages of three and four years, according to Robert Feldman, professor of psychology, at the University of Massachusetts at Amherst. "Kids are taught to do this, so, in a way, they are taught to be deceptive. A child is given a gift and is expected to smile whether he likes it or not. We call these social niceties, but it's really deceptive behavior," Feldman said in an interview.

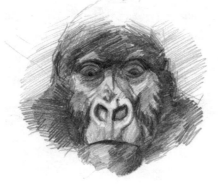

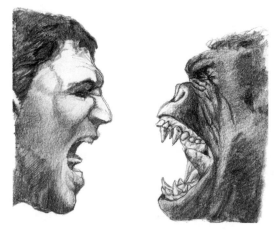

Alan Dixson in *The Natural History of the Gorilla*, asserts that gorillas stick out their tongues in apparent amazement, and yawn when stressed or uncertain—expressions shared by humans. Another facial expression is the so-called threat-bite, where a gorilla exposes its teeth, mouth open, to signal annoyance.

No matter how hard we may try to control our emotional expressions, we're slaves to our neurophysiology. ULCA psychiatrist Paul Ekman, who has studied facial expressions for decades, suggests that facial expressions of emotion—such as anger, fear, happiness, disgust—are involuntary. When we feel an emotion, signals are sent from our brain to the nerves of facial muscles. It happens in a microsecond. If emotion expressions are involuntary, then it would imply that they are more trustworthy, and direct.

Psychologist William Brown, of Dalhousie University (Nova Scotia), studied links between altruism and facial expressions, and found that altruistic people smile more than selfish people. He also found that altruists' smiles are symmetrical, and that phony smiles are less pronounced on the left side and last longer than "real" ones. Altruists also showed "concern furrows"—or a "heartfelt smile," which is extremely short and forms crow's feet around the eyes.

Examples of deception in gorillas have been recorded, but are quite rare. A free-ranging juvenile male built six nests— each in closer proximity to an infant—in what appeared to be an attempt to get closer in a deceptively sly manner. A captive female covered her smiling face with her hand 26 times while playing with a male playmate. Mothers "threat bite" their infants—an absurdly exaggerated threat—given that gorilla mothers don't hit or bite their infants.

Apart from these rare exceptions, most gorilla watchers have perceived that gorilla communication is dead honest.

GEORGE SCHALLER'S
FACIAL MOVEMENTS IN THE GORILLA AND MAN

gorilla*

- **Undisturbed, quiet state:** At rest, mouth closed and eyes "bland," inattentive.
- **Playface:** Mouth opened partially with the "corners drawn far back into a smile," teeth unclenched.
- **Annoyance:** Eyes "hard and fixed," head tipped slightly downward; lips often pursed and slightly parted. Forehead contracted and wrinkled in space between brow ridges.
- **Anger:** Eyes "hard and fixed" on the animal causing anger; exposed gums and teeth, and curled lips. Mouth either "half or entirely open, and the head is frequently tipped slightly down", accompanied by screams or roars.
- **Uneasiness:** Lips "characteristically pulled inward with the mouth remaining tightly compressed." Other signs include shifty eyes, lifted head, indirect stare.
- **Fear:** Almost indistinguishable from the anger face, but mouth opened a bit wider.

man**

- **Emotional expression:** Involuntary expressions caused by emotional states (happiness, sadness, anger, disgust, and so on).
- **Conversational signals:** Movements like raising an eyebrow or pressed lips, used as part of conversation to emphasize or react to words or thoughts.
- **False expressions:** A faked expression meant to look emotional. Can be detected by a trained eye.
- **Referential expressions:** Using emotional expressions to refer to an emotion being talked about. Not meant to be deceptive.
- **Emotional role-playing actions:** Described by psychologist and psychoanalyst Rainer Krause, these actions are emotional expressions made by someone feeling the emotions of a person he is depicting.

* Based on facial expressions of mountain gorillas described in George Schaller's classic *The Mountain Gorilla: Ecology and Behavior.*

* Based on Paul Ekman's *Should We Call it Expression or Communication?* Published in Innovations in Social Science Research.

"The eyes have a language of their own, being subtle
and silent mirrors of the mind, revealing constantly
changing patterns of emotion."
—George Schaller, *The Year of the Gorilla*

gestures

For all primates, there are appropriate gestures for most
situations. Choosing the right gesture depends on the
attentiveness of the receiver. Simone Pika and others of
the Max Planck Institute for Evolutionary Anthropology
(Leipzig, Germany), found that among western lowland
gorillas, silent gestures are used when the intended receiver
of the gesture exhibits a high degree of visual attention.
Auditory gestures are used when met with medium attention,
and tactile gestures are most frequently used in situations
involving low visual attention.

Of the 33 unique gestures Pika noted among western
lowland gorillas, most (16) were visual (arm shake, bow,
jump, stiff stance), 11 were tactile (embrace, hand touch
head, push, and gentle short touch), and only 6 were auditory
(chest beat, clap, stomp).

Does splashing water attract females?

Male western lowland gorillas have been spotted thrashing about in water in a display thought to intimidate other males and to attract females. A three-year study by Richard Parnell of the Wildlife Conservation Society of New York found that 14 different gorilla groups frequented swampy areas called "bais" in the Congolese Nouabale-Ndoki National Park to feed on aquatic plants. Parnell observed that solitary males did most of the splashing—which includes running or jumping into the water—and that their displays were directed nearly as much to females as they were directed to other solitary males.

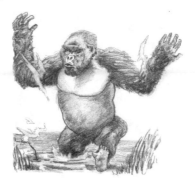

Pika and her team suggest that gorillas learn this complex alphabet of gestures by mimicking one another, repeating interactions, and being taught by their elders. She found that 80 percent of these gestures are used in three different contexts, and that all gestures in the repertoire are used when playing.

Simone Pika of the Max Planck Institute found that of 33 separate gestures western lowland gorillas use to communicate, 18 were visual, 11 were tactile and 6 were auditory.

koko, the signing gorilla

There's probably no better example of the learning capabilities and intelligence of gorillas than Koko, the renowned female lowland gorilla, who has a working vocabulary of some 1,000 signs (from American Sign Language) and understands some 2,000 words of spoken English.

Koko, born in 1971, was taught by developmental psychologist Francine "Penny" Patterson as an infant gorilla and, by age two, had learned 184 symbols. (This experiment was repeated by Patterson in her work with a male western

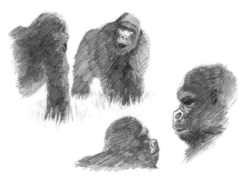

lowland gorilla named Michael.) Patterson's work with Koko—called Project Koko—led to the formation of the California-based *Gorilla Foundation*.

choose your grunts carefully
Grunting shows protest and annoyance, but it's also used to build consensus.

Consider mountain gorillas' "close-calls" (vocalizations made in close proximity), which are a sort of collective vote on when to end a resting or feeding period, according to University of California at Davis' Alexander Harcourt and Kelly Stewart.

Close-calls sessions are essentially open-air parliamentary votes. In the gorilla world, calling grunts sound different from response grunts. The "calls" mean "Are you ready to go?" and elicit response grunts meaning "Yes, I'm ready," which are quiet, calmly vocalized, "single" and "double" grunts. Grunts increase gradually in the final quarter of the resting period (culminating in a chorus), and 90 percent of these vocalizations are made when group members are still at rest. Adult males grunt the most, followed by adult females, then youngsters. When the chorus reaches a crescendo, the collective decision is finalized, and the group moves on.

In other studies, Harcourt and Kelly found that "non-syllabled" close-calls are used to appease others by announcing one's presence in a spirit of cooperation and submission. Double grunts can communicate the intention to begin an activity, and are more proactive and assertive. Grunts often determine social rank. For example, mid-ranked members make more double grunts to subordinates than to those ranked above them, and members use non-syllabled calls to dominant adult males more often than to lesser-ranked males.

CROSS-SPECIES GESTURING

Anthropologists at the Max Planck Institute found that western gorillas' gestures fell into three principal categories: visual, tactile, and auditory. Below are descriptions of each, and how they are curiously similar to the gestures of humans.

VISUAL used when gesturer has full visual attention of recipient of gesture.

TACTILE used when gesturer has partial visual attention of recipient.

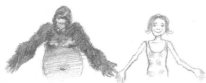

AUDITORY used when gesturer has little or no visual attention of the recipient.

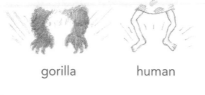

gorilla   human

displacement activity

Displacement activities are actions we take when torn between fighting and fleeing. For instance, consider road-rage behavior. The frustration of being stuck in bumper-to-bumper traffic is displaced by the incongruous activity of blowing the horn.

Primatologist George Schaller found displacement activities among mountain gorillas. They yawn when uneasy, or scratch their arms vigorously when in uncomfortable or threatening situations (while we scratch our heads). During chest-beating displays, gorillas pick up a piece of vegetation and feign to eat it. This activity, too, might serve the function of displacing the feeling of being caught between "fight-and-flight" urges.

Simone Pika of the Max Planck Institute found that of 33 separate gestures western lowland gorillas use to communicate, 18 were visual, 11 were tactile and 6 were auditory.

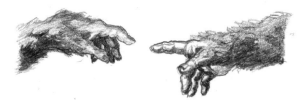

the right touch

"Haptic" is the word nonverbal communication researchers use to describe communication through touch.

Humans communicate nonverbally to varying degrees, but, compared to gorillas, fall more on the "touch avoidance" end of the spectrum. Of course, our behavior varies from culture to culture. In Britain and the United States, kissing as a greeting is far less common than, say, in France. Handshakes will do in some cultures, but hugs are customary in others. Despite the cultural variance, we're still eons away from the gorillas in communicating through touch.

According to Max Planck Institute's Simone Pika's western lowland gorilla study, mentioned earlier, tactile gestures are the most flexible, and are used in the most contexts.

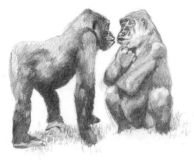

The following tactile gestures were the most common:

Touch (gentle touch with hands or feet, lasting
        less than five seconds);
Grab (holding on to another animal);
Punch (a short thrust with knuckles, finger
        or fist);
Slap (running, then slapping with open palm)

Other touching includes hugging, kissing (touching lips),
and stroking. Social grooming could count as tactile
communication, too, which, on the surface, is done to
remove debris and parasites from another's hair. But it
can also be a bonding and trust-building activity between
mothers and infants, younger gorillas, and youngsters
grooming silverbacks.

Humans seem to under-use tactile gestures, with the most common (handshake, slap on the back, mock kiss without lips touching face) being our ritualized greetings. Some psychologists feel that we're built to receive and give more touch, and that this explains the health benefits of having pets—and even explains the satisfaction of playfully throwing a pillow at somebody.

signs of subordination

Far from being ignoble or humiliating, submissive behavior amongst gorillas plays an important peacekeeping role within the group and between groups. Submissive gestures are used to cool heads when threatened, signaling lack of interest in

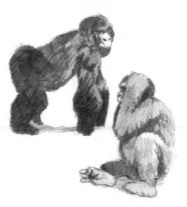

engaging in confrontation. Some examples of submissive behavior are the giving a sideways glance, or turning the head to avoid making eye contact.

Physical cowering can be interpreted as a peacekeeping mannerism, rather than a sign of cowardice. Gorillas cower by leaning at the waist, or placing their hands on their heads. We use non-threatening stylized gestures, too—nodding, bowing, tipping the hat, or shaking our head back and forth.

As mentioned earlier, gorilla subordinates can appease by chorusing. Harcourt and Stewart found that mountain gorillas make a chorus (exchange of frequent quiet calls in close proximity) when finding a good feeding area, or when embracing. This chorusing or use of non-syllable vocalizations during feeding and movement may serve to avert competition or antagonism with higher-ranking members or outside groups.

Physical cowering can be interpreted as a peacekeeping mannerism rather than a sign of cowardice.

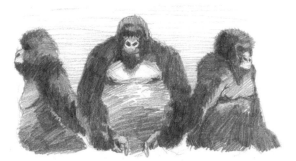

making up

Female and males gorillas can groom and use non-threatening vocalizations to make up after a fight (i.e., post-conflict reconciliation), but generally don't make as much of a fuss as other primates.

But according to UCLA's Joan Silk, reconciliation isn't exactly necessary. She asserts that there is no evidence that peaceful post-conflict behavior affects long-term relationships between bickering individuals. The major exception is that females tend to make up with the silverback by grooming or making non-syllabled or "appeasement" vocalizations. It is puzzling that female gorillas do not typically reconcile after a fight with one another, given that related and unrelated females can have extremely close relationships. This might be due to the fact that gorilla females are, in general, on the same hierarchical level, and, therefore, don't feel the need to make special efforts to protect relationships other than those with a higher-ranking individual (such as the silverback or other adult males).

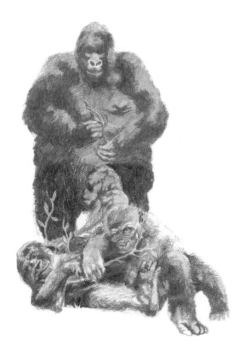

Building effective body language is crucial to becoming a welcomed and solid group member.

body (language) building

For gorillas, being fluent at reading and interpreting body language could mean the difference between moving up the social ladder, or being ostracized as a loner. Not providing the young with all the confidence and care that touching seems to engender could mean a troubled youth later.

Not taking a silverback's cold, hard stare with the grave seriousness it merits could have serious consequences. Building body language, suffice it to say, is crucial to being a solid and welcome group member.

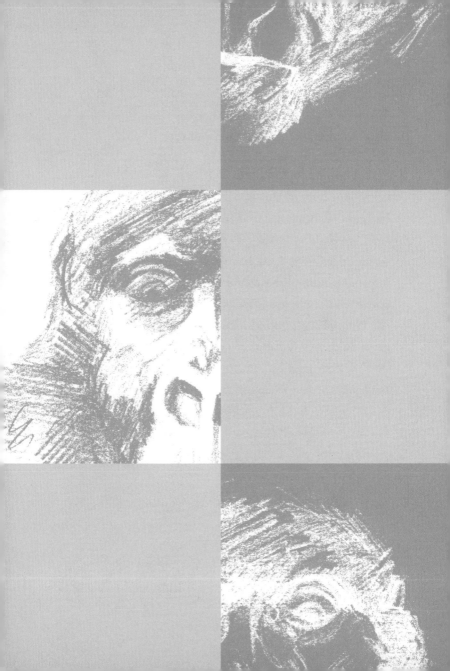

chapter six

gorilla nomenclature and species characteristics

There are two main gorilla species—the western gorilla and the eastern gorilla—with populations spanning eight countries across central and western equatorial Africa. Within these species are five subspecies. These include the **western lowland gorilla,** which is the most common gorilla in zoos, and has the largest wild population of all gorilla species—and the **mountain gorilla,** the animals studied by Dian Fossey, and the rarest of the two species. This chapter is a brief primer on the gorilla subspecies—their population, habitat, physical traits and on discovery by humans.

the discoverers

The first gorilla to be documented as a newly discovered species was a western lowland gorilla found in Gabon by

Americans Thomas Staughton Savage and Jeffries Wyman in 1847. They assigned the animal, based on a skull and skeletal remains, the scientific name of TROGLODYTES GORILLA.

Captain Robert von Beringe, a member of the German colonial force in Africa, is attributed with writing the first account of a living mountain gorilla. In 1902, von Beringe, who was interested in African wildlife and plant life, happened upon mountain gorillas while traveling through the Virunga mountain range. Two of the gorillas were shot and fell into a volcanic crater. One was retrieved, with some parts sent to Berlin, and identified by Paul Matschie. The mountain gorilla's scientific name, GORILLA BERINGEI BERINGEI, was named after the captain.

Austrian Rudolf Grauer, an African enthusiast and collector, made several African visits from 1907 to 1911. On his last trip, he shot a gorilla near Lake Tanganjika, and brought back its hide and skull to Europe, where it was indentified—again by Paul Matschie—as a new gorilla species. The eastern lowland gorilla, GORILLA BERINGEI GRAUERI, is named after Grauer.

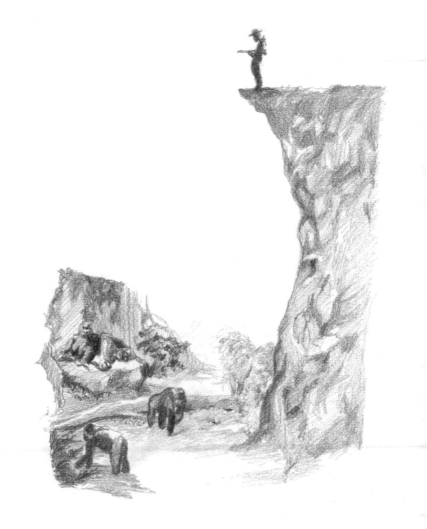

GORILLA TIMELINE: PREHISTORIC

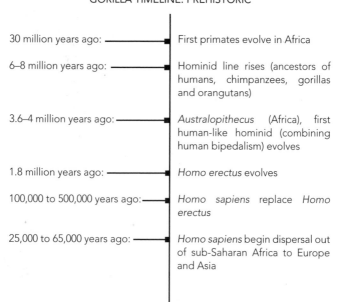

30 million years ago: — First primates evolve in Africa

6–8 million years ago: — Hominid line rises (ancestors of humans, chimpanzees, gorillas and orangutans)

3.6–4 million years ago: — *Australopithecus* (Africa), first human-like hominid (combining human bipedalism) evolves

1.8 million years ago: — *Homo erectus* evolves

100,000 to 500,000 years ago: — *Homo sapiens* replace *Homo erectus*

25,000 to 65,000 years ago: — *Homo sapiens* begin dispersal out of sub-Saharan Africa to Europe and Asia

GORILLA TIMELINE: MODERN

1847:	First recorded identification of lowland gorilla: Thomas Staughton Savage and Jeffries (Gabon)
1849:	Charles Darwin publishes *On the Origin of Species*
1902:	Captain Robert von Beringe first identifies the mountain gorilla
1921:	Carl Akeley (of The American Museum of Natural History) leads pioneering expedition to Mt. Mikeno in the Virungas
1930:	Robert Yerkes founds Yerkes National Primate Research Center
March 23, 1933:	*King Kong* premieres at Grauman's Chinese Theatre in Hollywood
Dec. 22, 1956:	Colo is the world's first western lowland gorilla born in captivity (Columbus Zoo)
1959:	George Schaller begins researching the mountain gorilla in the Virungas
1967:	Dian Fossey founds the Karisoke Research Center in Rwanda
July 4, 1971:	Koko the gorilla is born
December 31, 1984:	Massa, oldest known gorilla, at 54, dies at Philadelphia Zoo
August 2009:	A census finds that there are about 125,000 more western lowland gorillas than previously thought in the swampy forests of northern Republic of Congo

THE FOUR (OR FIVE?) GORILLA SUBSPECIES

The western species has two subspecies: the western lowland and Cross River gorillas. The eastern species has three subspecies: the mountain, eastern lowland and Bwindi Forest gorillas. (As research continues on precisely how Bwindi gorillas [who live in the Bwindi Impenetrable Forest National Park in southern Uganda] differ from other gorilla subspecies, there is not yet complete agreement among researchers and primatologists over whether this animal ought to be classified as a distinct subspecies.)

Regarding the original nomenclature of the word gorilla, whether myth or folklore, it's attributed to Hanno, a sixth-century Greek explorer who used the Greek word gorillai, meaning hairy women, which the local peoples in northwestern Africa supposedly called gorillas.

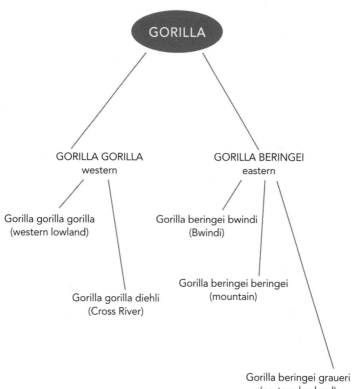

where they live

While the traditional gorilla ranges have changed profoundly (that is, gotten smaller and more fragmentized), largely due to man's activities, the basic pockets of habitat are along the Equator in central and west Africa. The much-studied mountain gorillas live in the rich mountain rainforests straddling Rwanda, Uganda, and the Democratic Republic of Congo (DRC, and formerly Zaire). Generally, eastern lowland gorillas live in eastern DRC, and Uganda, and western lowland gorillas live in western Africa and the Congo River Basin (this area includes Gabon, Cameroon, Nigeria, Central African Republic, and western DRC).

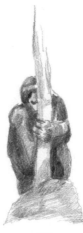

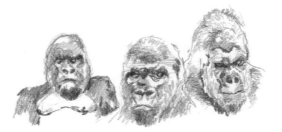

vital statistics

The following sections provide at-a-glance particulars on the major gorilla species, and how they differ not only in physical characteristics, but also in their habitats and estimated population numbers. Keep in mind that while there has been considerable research carried out on these subspecies— particularly the mountain gorilla—the information that follows has been compiled from a number of various studies and sources. Owing to the profoundly difficult tasks of collecting such information, like population numbers, there are divergent estimates, and hence, the ranges, averages and approximations present herein. Also, note that, in the spirit of simplification, only the three most highly studied gorilla species are featured here. Some estimates are likely more accurate than others, depending on the depth of research.

MOUNTAIN GORILLA

- **Scientific name:** Gorilla beringei beringei
- **Average male height:** 5'8"
- **Average** male arm span: 7'6"
- **Average male weight:** 343 lbs.
- **Population estimate in the wild:** About 325 mountain gorillas; about 325 Bwindi gorillas (considered by some as its own subspecies).
- **Average group size:** 9
- **Diet:** Chiefly green plant parts (i.e., pith, leaves, stem, shoots).Favorites include bamboo shoots, gallium, thistles, celery and nettles.
- **Habitat:** Mountain forest in Uganda, Rwanda, Democratic Republic of Congo. Live in altitudes of up to 3,900 meters. Much studied in the Virunga Volcanoes National Park and the Karisoke Research Station in Rwanda, and the Bwindi Impentrable Forest in Uganda.
- **Distinguishing physical characteristics:** Fur is black, and longer and thicker than western lowlands, particularly on the arms and around the face. Massive teeth and jaws.

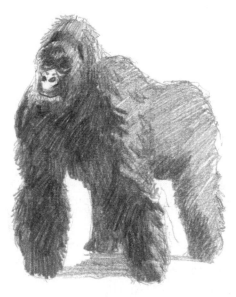

MOUNTAIN GORILLA

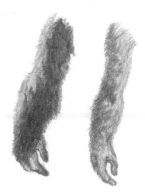

The mountain gorilla's longer, shaggier and thicker undercoat provides better protection against the cold and wet climate in the mountain forests.

EASTERN LOWLAND GORILLA

- **Scientific name:** Gorilla beringei graueri
- **Average male height:** 5'9"
- **Arm male arm span:** 7'6"
- **Average male weight:** 360 lbs.
- **Population estimate in the wild:** About 4,000–10,000
- **Average group size:** 9–10
- **Diet:** Fruits, seeds, green leafy plants (shoots, pith, stem and bark).
- **Habitat:** Tropical lowland and forests in Uganda and eastern part of the Democratic Republic of Congo and Uganda.
- **Distinguishing physical characteristics:** Long, narrow face, short hair on the back, and longer hair on other parts of the body.

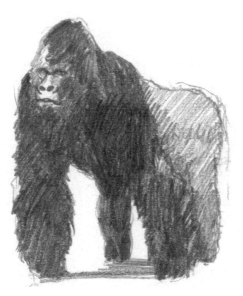

EASTERN LOWLAND GORILLA

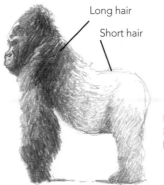

Long hair

Short hair

Eastern Lowlands are characterized by the short hair on their backs.

WESTERN LOWLAND GORILLA

- **Scientific name:** Gorilla gorilla gorilla
- **Average male height:** 5'6"
- **Average male arm span:** 7'8"
- **Average male weight:** 307 lbs.
- **Population estimate in the wild:** About 150,000
- **Average group size:** 9
- **Diet:** Mostly fruit when in season; in dry season, mostly green plant parts, seeds, and tree bark. Favorites include plants belonging to the ginger and arrowroot families.
- **Habitat:** Primary forest, and marshy forest clearings, known as bias. Live in the rainforests of Nigeria, Gabon, Cameroon, Central African Republic, and western Democratic Republic of Congo.
- **Distinguishing physical characteristics:** Brownish hair, shorter and thinner than mountain gorillas. Pronounced brow ridge. Ears seem smaller in relation to head, compared to mountain gorillas. Adult males' heads look conical, due to large bony crests on top. Wider and larger skull and broad nose. Big toe is spread wider than the other four toes.

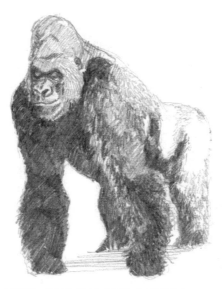

WESTERN LOWLAND GORILLA

Western lowlands' big toe is spread further from the second digit, compared to other subspecies.

A SHORT LIFE HISTORY

- **Birth:** Typically lasts less than one hour, but difficult births can last up to three days
- **Years 1-3:** Infants (nursed for at least two years)
- **Years 3-6:** Juveniles (learning all requirements of foraging, nest-building, group behavior, gender roles)
- **Year 8:** Female start to become sexually mature. Males are called blackbacks until they mature into silverbacks, around age 13–15, and breed.
- **Years approximately 30–45:** Old age. Ailments such as arthritis, affecting bones in hands and feet, tooth loss from periodontis makes feeding difficult, traveling and foraging are hard. Other group members adjust ranging to accommodate the aged.
- **End of years:** Group members abandon the aged only when death is clearly imminent, or the aged retreat off by themselves to die.

REPRODUCTION—SOME BASIC FACTS

- Females ovulate at 8 to 10 years old
- **Hormone cycle in females:** 26–32 days
- Come into estrus at mid-cycle, lasting 1–4 days
- Period lasts for two days
- During estrus, females approach males and females more frequently
- **Average pregnancy period:** 257 days
- Mothers give birth approximately every three to four years
- Twin births occur as frequently as with humans
- **Average weight of newborn (western lowland):** 2,200 grams, compared to 3,300 grams in humans
- **Largest known number of surviving offspring from one mother:** 6 (from a mountain gorilla)

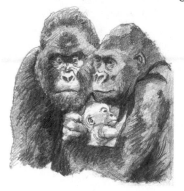

LEAVING HOME

As indicated in the chart below, most gorillas leave their natal group when adolescents. Males will join other groups, or go it alone and start new ones, or, in rare cases, co-join with other male-only groups. Nearly three-quarters of females, on the other hand, leave their natal group in search of joining a male or an established group. These common female departures to other unrelated groups, perhaps not coincidentally, limit inbreeding.

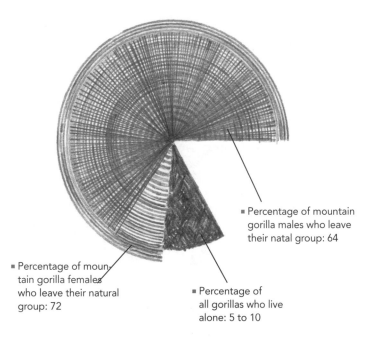

■ Percentage of mountain gorilla males who leave their natal group: 64

■ Percentage of mountain gorilla females who leave their natural group: 72

■ Percentage of all gorillas who live alone: 5 to 10

HOW GORILLAS SPEND THEIR DAY

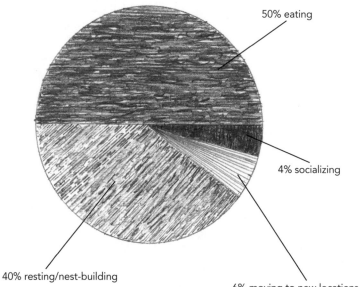

50% eating

4% socializing

40% resting/nest-building

6% moving to new locations

How does a gorilla spend its day? Pretty much the way we might like to—if we could. Half the day is spent eating, and the rest is spent looking for ways to rest. A sliver of the day's pie is spent roaming about to find new places to eat and sleep, and the remainder is spent socializing.

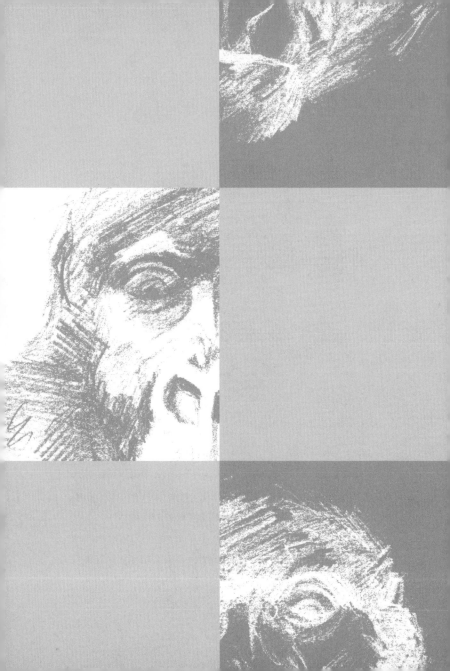

chapter seven

saving the gorilla

Up until this chapter, we've focused on the good news about gorillas and how looking more closely at these remarkable animals might prompt us to look more closely at ourselves.

This final section surveys the bad news—how desperately threatened the gorilla and its habitat have become over the decades. Indeed, there have been great resources and efforts dedicated to saving the gorilla—but much more clearly needs to be done.

We need a shift in thinking and heart that forces a true belief that man and wildlife can, and should, live together in harmony. Beyond the moral soundness of this argument, it is clear that efforts directed at saving endangered wildlife are, in and of themselves, efforts to save mankind as well.

At the end of this chapter are resources that can guide readers to reputable, information-rich organizations mostly committed to wildlife conservation and research. Plus, there are a few simple, but vital, suggestions of how ordinary people can help save the gorilla.

threats

A combination of pressures and threats have placed all five of the gorilla species on the endangered species list (the Mountain and Cross River gorillas are "critically endangered"). The encroachment on their sensitive habitat and ecosystem—and assault upon them directly—usually points to one culprit: man. Other than indigenous pathogens and species-specific illness (and, perhaps the leopard, the gorilla's only non-human predator), diminished gorilla populations are a product of human activity.

The Primate Specialist Group of the IUCN and Conservation International estimate that about 20 percent of wild primates could be wiped out in the next 20 years unless strong actions are carried out to offset or remove current threats.

While much has been achieved to protect the habitats of the gorillas and great apes, threats still persist in the form of deforestation, bushmeat hunters, human settlement, and disease (in particular the Zaire strain of the Ebola virus).

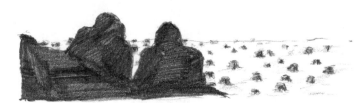

Here are brief overviews of the gravest threats impacting the well-being of the gorilla and its traditional habitat.

■ LOGGING AND DEFORESTATION   Large bands of tropical forests have been disturbed or destroyed across equatorial Africa due to mining, logging, human settlement, and agriculture. Despite efforts by governments and conservation groups to limit deforestation in sensitive areas, the damage continues. The World Wildlife Fund estimates that in the Congo River Basin (the world's second largest tropical forest), nearly four million acres is ravaged each year. If deforestation continues unabated, an estimated two-thirds of this rich and important ecosystem will vanish in 50 years.

In Cameroon, 60 percent of the surviving 42 million acres of forest are already being exploited. Deforestation is particularly threatening small pockets of habitat, such as the 164-square-mile Virunga National Park, home to

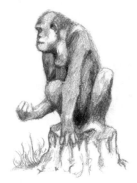

almost half of the world's mountain gorilla population. By the summer of 2004, approximately ten percent of the park was illegally deforested. Slash-and-burning of forests not only scars the fragile biosystem and high biomass areas used by the great apes, but also contributes significantly to carbon dioxide emissions in the atmosphere, which contribute to the greenhouse effect.

Beyond the direct damage to the habitat caused by deforestation, the roads required for logging and mining usher in a host of other problems, such as bushmeat poachers and hunters, human settlement and contact, described further below. The United Nations' Great Apes Survival Project (GRASP) has estimated that, at current levels of deforestation, less than one-tenth of existing great ape habitats will remain undisturbed by 2030.

■ BUSHMEAT HUNTING/POACHING Slaughtering gorillas for meat occurs on an alarming scale. Gorillas are believed to be illegally killed by poachers and hunters, many of whom use logging roads to access the animals. Other deaths occur when gorillas are caught in snares set for duikers (forest antelope). According to The International Primate Protection League (IPPL), 400 to 600 gorillas are killed annually in the DRC alone, with estimates of as many as 2,000 in total across Africa anually. A 2001 survey by primatologist Alastair McNeilage, of the protected Bwindi Forest, found considerable human distburbance: 62 snares, 34 human trails, 3 pitsawing sites, and 21 fireplaces.

Gorillas are being hunted in increasing numbers in Cameroon and DRC. Hunters smoke gorilla meat to make it less identifiable from other bushmeat when sold in markets or to village restaurants. Gorilla meat is believed to be shipped to villages on logging trucks, according to the IPPL.

The prices are shocking: a smoked gorilla can fetch about US$40 for the hunters, and a chimp, US$20. Given that a significant numbers of local inhabitants near gorilla habitats rely on bushmeat as a traditional source of protein, it is particularly difficult to enforce gorilla poaching.

■ EBOLA   In the last decade, roughly 30 percent—or tens of thousands—of the western lowland gorilla population are estimated to have been lost due to the deadly Ebola virus. Since 2001, researchers conservatively estimate that about 5,500 gorilla deaths in the Republic of Congo alone have been attributed to outbreaks of the so-called Zaire strain of the Ebola virus, which kills victims, including chimps and humans, in about a week. About 90 percent of Gabon's gorilla population is estimated to have vanished due to Ebola.

While researchers have tried injecting Ebola vaccines, it is not an easy task, and more research is needed on how best to administer them (by darts or orally) and on the vaccines' effectiveness. It is also time consuming and costly to protect significant numbers of gorillas. More field research and capital investment is needed to carry out a meaningful Ebola vaccination program to prevent more widespread infection and death.

■ OTHER DISEASE   Great apes are highly susceptible to human disease, and can catch a long list of illnesses through close contact with man or from domesticated animals living too close to gorilla ranges. Almost anything touched by man—clothing, toilet paper, handkerchiefs, cigarette butts— can spread bacteria and viruses via respiratory infection or through fecal-oral infection.

DISEASES GORILLAS CAN CATCH

Common cold
Pneumonia
Influenza
Hepatitis
Smallpox
Chicken pox
Bacterial meningitis
Tuberculosis
Measles
Rubella

Mumps
Yellow fever
Encephalomyocarditis
Ebola fever

Parasitic Diseases
Malaria
Schistomiasis
Giardiases
Filariasis

Stress caused by man and his activities can also weaken gorillas' immunity, making them more vulnerable to disease and illness. Alpha herpes and scabies, for example, are stress-related conditions gorillas have contracted. Finally, gorillas who feed on human dumps, or on cultivated land on the fringes of the parks, can also get infected with human and domesticated animal illnesses.

civil war/unrest

In the last several decades, civil war and political unrest near and within gorilla habitats have left scars on these ecosystems and have, at times, hobbled conservation efforts. In the 1980s, for example, before Rwanda's brutal civil strife, ecotourism generated significant profits, aiding Rwanda's economy, the local population, and the building of a sustainable gorilla conservation program.

Other flashpoints over the years, including the Democratic Republic of Congo (DRC) and Uganda, have made gorilla tourism harrowingly dangerous destinations. The effects of civil war on gorilla habitats are widespread and include the collapse of monitoring illegal activities such as settlement and trespassing within the parks, bushmeat

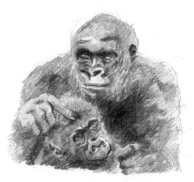

hunting, even the murdering of park staff, not to mention plummeting revenue from reduced ecotourism.

saving the gorilla

Apart from going back to school and getting a doctorate or moving to Rwanda, there are significant ways to prevent further encroachment upon, and threats to, the gorilla and its habitats and to endangered wildlife in general.

individual donation

The most obvious way to help is to make a donation to a conservation group of your choice. This chapter includes a list of some of these. Write a check yourself, or think of a creative alternative way to contribute (ask people to make a donation in your name to an organization of your choice in lieu of a wedding, birthday or anniversary present).

grassroots fundraising

Organize a fundraising drive or a raffle in your neighborhood, workplace, or place of worship. Use a small percentage of the money raised to buy all contributors a premium thank-you gift. Remember to confirm if contributions are tax-deductible, and make this known to contributors.

spreading the word

To help raise awareness of the endangered African rain forests and lowland forests (and wildlife conservation in general), share related information about reputable conservation and research groups with education and con-servation initiatives at schools, in the workplace, with boy and girl scout troops, summer camps, and other organizations.

be a responsible ecotourist

Though gorilla watching can be prohibitively expensive, the lucky few who can afford the time, money, and arduous journey to do so are blessed. The costs do much to support the livelihoods of many locals who have chosen to work to preserve the sensitive ecosystem and the fragile populations literally in their backyards. But only by making sure that all ecotourism protocols are strictly followed, will your dollars be well spent. Tour groups will have rules that vary, but below are some basic ones that are generally accepted for all who enter the gorilla's world:

- Do not visit the gorillas if you have a contagious illness
- Do not touch the gorillas—keep at least 20 feet away
- Do not leave anything behind (trash, food, clothing, toilet paper)
- Limit your group number to about a half-dozen ecotourists
- Use tours that visit gorilla groups only once a stay
- Keep visits to less than one hour
- Do nothing to provoke a gorilla (prolonged eye contact, sudden movements)
- Do not use flash photography

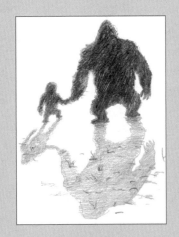

resources

- Africa Conservancy, www.africaconservancy.org
- The African Conservation Foundation, www.africanconservation.org
- African Wildlife Foundation, www.awf.org
- Association of Zoos & Aquariums, www.aza.org
- The Cameroon Wildlife Aid Fund, www.cwaf.org
- The Convention on International Trade in Endangered Species, www.cites.org
- Conservation International, www.conservation.org
- The Dian Fossey Gorilla Fund, www.gorillafund.org
- European Association of Zoos and Aquaria, www.eaza.net
- Forest Conservation Links Page, http//forests.org/links/
- The Gorilla Organization, www.gorillas.org
- International Gorilla Conservation Programme, www.mountaingorillas.org
- IPPL (International Primate Protection League), www.ippl.org

- The IUCN Red List, www.redlist.org
- The Jane Goodall Institute, www.janegoodall.org
- Mountain Gorilla Conservation Fund, www.saveagorilla.org
- The Mountain Gorilla Protection Project, www.informatics.org/gorilla
- The North Carolina Zoo, http//nczoo.org
- The Pan African Sanctuary Alliance (PASA),
  www.panafricanprimates.org
- The Rainforest Action Network, www.ran.org
- The Rainforest Alliance, www.rainforest-alliance.org
- The Rainforest Foundation, www.savetherainforest.org
- San Diego Zoological Society, www.sandiegozoo.org
- The Wildlife Conservation Society, www.wcs.org
- The Wisconsin National Primate Research Center,
  www.primate.wisc.edu
- The World Wild Fund, www.worldwildlife.org
- The Wasmoeth Wildlife Foundation, www.wasmoethwildlife.org
- The Wildlife Protector's Fund/Gorilla Foundation, www.gorilla.org

bushmeat sites

- Biosynergy Institute, www.bushmeat.net
- The Ape Alliance, www.4apes.com
- Bushmeat Crisis Task Force, www.bushmeat.org
- GRASP, www.unep.org/grasp

selected sources by chapter

The author acknowledges the following body of literature that both directly and indirectly contributed to the depth of this work, and gratefully acknowledges the spirit and rigor which the authors cited have demonstrated in their respective, varied fields.

chapter 1: growing up

Ed. Robbins, Martha M., Sicotte, Pascale, Stewart, Kelly J, *Mountain Gorillas: Three decades of research at Karisoke*. Cambridge, UK: Cambridge University Press, 2001. N.B.: The following chapters were useful for this chapter: Clever hands: The food-processing skills of mountain gorillas, Byrne, Richard W., (pages 293-314) and "Development of infant independence from the mother in wild mountain gorillas" by Alison Fletcher (pages 153-182).

Fields, Jason. "Children's Living Arrangements and Characteristics" *Current Population Reports*. Washington, DC.: U.S. Census Bureau, 2003.

Fossey, Dian, *Gorillas in the Mist*, London: Penguin, 1985.

Maestripieri, Dario, et al., "Mother-Infant Interactions in Western Lowland Gorillas (Gorilla gorilla gorilla): Spatial Relationships, Communication, and Opportunities for Social Learning," *Journal of Comparative Psychology*, Vol. 116, No. 3, 219-227 (2002).

Maestripieri, Dario, "Parent-Offspring Conflict in Primates", *International Journal of Primatology*, Volume 23, No. 4, August 2002.

Pika, Simone, et al., "Gestural Communication in Young Gorillas (Gorilla gorilla): Gesture Repertoire, Learning, and Use", *American Journal of Primatology* 60: 95-111 (2003).

Schaller, George B., The Mountain Gorilla, Chicago: University of Chicago Press, 1963.

Schaller, George B., *The Year of the Gorilla*, Chicago: The University of Chicago Press, 1964.

Sicotte, Pascale, "Interpositions in Conflicts between Males in Bimale Groups of Mountain Gorillas," *Folia Primatologica*, 1995, 65:14-24.

Stewart, Kelly J., "Social Relationships of Immature Gorillas and Silver-backs, The Birth of a Wild Mountain Gorilla (Gorilla gorilla bereingei)," *Primates*, 18(4): 965-976, October 1977.

chapter 2: family ties

Fossey, Dian, Gorillas in the Mist, London: Penguin Books, 1985.

Klinker, Joan, "Early Childhood Excellence Insights," Wisconsin's Early Childhood Excellence Initiative, University of Wisconsin-Extension, August 2002, No. 14.

Maestripieri, Dario, et al., "Mother-Infant Interactions in Western Low-land Gorillas (Gorilla gorilla gorilla): Spatial Relationships, Communication, and Opportunities for Social Learning," *Journal of Comparative Psychology*, 2002, Vol. 116, No. 3, 219-227.

Maestripieri, Dario, "Parent-Offspring Conflict in Primates," *International Journal of Primatology*, Vol. 23, No. 4, August 2002.

Robbins, Martha M., Sicotte, Pascale and Stewart, Kelly J. *Mountain Gorillas: Three Decades of Research at Karisoke.* Cambridge, UK: Cambridge University Press, 2001.

Schaller, George B., *The Mountain Gorilla*, Chicago and London: University of Chicago Press, 1963.

Schaller, George B., *The Year of the Gorilla*, Chicago and London: The University of Chicago Press, 1964.

Schore, Allan, N., "The Effects of a Secure Attachment Regulation on Right Brain Development, Affect Regulation, 150 and Infant Mental Health", *Infant Mental Health Journal*, 22, 7-66 (2001).

Sicotte, Pascale, "Interpositions in Conflicts between Males in Bi-male Groups of Mountain Gorillas," *Folia Primatologica,*; 65: 14-24 (1995).

chapter 3: the silverback

Bennis, Warren, "The Secrets of Great Groups," Leader to Leader, Winter 1997, pp. 29-33.

Bradley, Brenda, et al., "Dispersed Male Networks in Western Gorillas," *Current Biology*, Vol. 14, 510-513, 2004.

Doran, Diane M., McNeilage, Alastair, "Gorilla Ecology and Behavior," *Evolutionary Anthropology*, 6, 1998, 120-131.

Harcourt, A. H., Stewart, K.J., "Functions of Wild Gorilla 'Close' Calls: Repertoire, Context, and Interspecific Comparison," Behaviour, 124 (1-2) 1993.

Harcourt, A. H., Stewart, K.J., "Functions of Wild Gorilla 'Close' Calls. Repertoire, Context, and Interspecific Comparison," *Behaviour*, 133, 827-845, 1996.

House, Robert J., Aditya, Ram N., "The Social Scientific Study of Leadership: Quo Vadis?," *Journal of Management*, 1997, Vol. 23, No. 3, 409-473.

Margulis,S.W., Whitham, J.C., Ogorzalek,K.,"Silverback Male Presence and group Stability in Gorillas (Gorilla gorilla gorilla)," Folio Primatologica, 2003, 74: 92-96.

Riggio, Ronald E. "Assessment of Basic Social Skills," *Journal of Personality and Social Psychology*. 1986, Vol. 51, No. 3, 649-660.

Riggio, R.E., Zimmerman, J.,"Social Skills and Interpersonal Relationships: Influences on Social Support and Support Seeking," In W.H. Jones (D. Perlman (Eds.), *Advances in Personal Relationships*, Vol. 2, pages 133-155, 1991.

Riggio, Ronald, and E. Charisms, *Encyclopedia of Mental Health*, Vol. 1," Academic Press, 1998, pp 387-395.

Robbins, Martha, "Variation in the Social System of mountain Gorillas: The Male Perspective," from *Mountain Gorillas, Three Decades of Research at Karisoke*, Cambridge, UK: Cambridge University Press, 2001.

Schaller, George, *The Mountain Gorilla: Ecology and Behavior,* London: The University of Chicago Press, 1963.

Sicotte, Pascale, "Inter-Group Encounters and Female Transfer in Mountain Gorillas: Influence of Group composition on Male Behavior," *American Journal of Primatology*, 30: 21-36 (1993).

Silk, Joan B. "Practice Random Acts of Aggression and Senseless Acts of Intimidation: The Logic of Status Contests in Social Groups," *Evolutionary Anthropology* 11: 221-225 (2002).

Silk, Joan B. "The Function of Peaceful Post-Conflict Contacts Among Primates," *Primates*, 38(3): 265-279, July 1997.

Silk, Joan, et al., "Cheap Talk When Interests Conflict," *Animal Behaviour*, 2000, 59, 423-432.

Stewart, Kelly J., Harcourt, Alexander H. "Gorillas' Vocalizations During Rest Periods: Signals of Impending Departure?," *Behaviour*, 130 (1-2) 1994.

Watts, David P. "Agonistic Interventions in Wild Mountain Gorilla Groups," *Behaviour, 134, 23-57.*

chapter 4: eating out

Byrne, Richard W., Byrne, Jennifer M.E., "Complex Leaf-Gathering Skills of Mountain Gorillas (Gorilla g. beringei): Variability and Standardization," American Journal of Primatology, 31: 241-261 (1993).

Dixson, A.F. PhD, The Natural History of the Gorilla, London: Weidenfeld and Nicolson, 1981.

Ed. Robbins, Martha M., Sicotte, Pascale and Stewart, Kelly J., Mountain Gorillas: Three Decades of Research at Karisoke, Cambridge, UK: Cambridge University Press, 2001.

NB. The following chapters were useful in this chapter:

—Feeding ecology of free-ranging mountain gorilla (Gorilla gorilla beringei), D. Fossey and A.H. Harcourt, pages 415-447.
—Feeding and ranging behaviour of a Mountain Gorilla Group, (Gorilla gorilla beringei) in the Tshibinda-Kahuzi Region (Zaire), Allan G. Goodall, pages 449-479.
—Clever hands: The food-processing skills of mountain gorillas, Byrne, Richard W., pages 293-314.
—Diet and habitat use of two mountain gorilla groups in contrasting habitats in the Virungas, McNeilage, Alistair, pages 293-314.

Ed. Clutton-Brock, T.H., *Primate Ecology: Studies of feeding and ranging behavior in lemurs, monkeys and apes*, London: 146 Academic Press Inc., 1977.

Food, Nutrition, and the Prevention of Cancer: A global perspective, Washington, D.C.: World Cancer Research Fund/American Institute for Cancer Research, 1997.

Fossey, Dian, *Gorillas in the Mist*, London: Penguin, 1985.

Goldberg, Gail. *Plants: Diet and Health. The report of the British Nutrition Foundation Task Force*, London: Blackwell, 2003.

Jenkins, David J.A., et. al., "A Dietary Portfolio Approach to Cholesterol Reduction: Combined Effects of Plant Sterols, Vegetable Proteins, and Viscous Fibers in Hypercholesterlemia," *Metabolism*, Vol. 51, No 12 (December), 2002, pages 1596-1604.

Jenkins, David J.A., MD, et. al., "Effects of a Dietary Portfolio of Cholesterol-Lowering Foods vs Lovastatin on Serum Lipids and C-reactive Protein," JAMA, July 23/30, 2003—Vol. 290, No. 4.

Jenkins, David, et. al., "Effect on Blood Lipids of very high intakes of Fiber in Diets Low in Saturated Fat and Cholesterol," *The New England Journal of Medicine*, Vol. 329: 21-26, July 1, 1993, No. 1.

Krauss, Ronald M. et al., *AHA Dietary Guidelines: Revision 2000: A Statement for Healthcare Professionals From the Nutrition Committee of the American Heart Association*, American Heart Association, 2000.

Lupton, Joanne R., PhD, "Is Fiber Protective Against Colon Cancer? Where the Research is Leading Us," *Nutrition*, Vol. 16, No. 7/8, 2000.

Mahaney, William C., et al., "Mountain Geophagy: A Possible Seasonal Behavior for Dealing with the Effects of Dietary Changes," *International Journal of Primatology*, Vol. 16, 1995, No.3.

Mariana-Costantini, Aldo, MD, "Natural and Cultural Influences on the Evolution of the Human Diet: Background of the Multifactorial Processes That Shaped the Eating Habits of Western Societies," *Nutrition*, Vol. 16, No. 7/8, 2000.

Milton, Katherine, "Eating What Comes Naturally: An Examination of Some Differences Between the Dietary Components of Humans and Wild Primates." A presentation prepared for The Origins and Evolution of Human Diet, 14th International Congress of Anthropological and Ethnological Sciences, July 26-August 1, 1998, Williamsburg, Virginia, USA.

Milton, Katherine, PhD, "Back to Basics: Why Foods of Wild Primates Have relevance for Modern Human Health", *Nutrition,* Vol. 16, Numbers 7/8, 2000.

Milton, Katherine, PhD, "Nutritional Characteristics of Wild Primate Foods: Do the Diets of Our Closest Living Relatives Have Lessons for Us?," *Nutrition*, Vol. 15, No. 6, 1999.

Nishihara, Tomoaki, "Feeding Ecology of Western Lowland gorillas in the Nouabale-Ndoki National Park, Congo," *Primates*, 36(2): 151-168, April 1995.

Pi, Sabater, Jorge, "Contribution to the Study of Alimentation of Lowland Gorillas in the Natural State, in Rio Muni, Republic of Equatorial Guinea (West Africa)," *Primates*; 19(1):183-204, January 1977.

Plumptre, A.J., "The Chemical Composition of Montane Plants and its Influence on the Diet of the Large Mammalian Herbivores in the Parc National des Volcans, Rwanda," *Journal of Zoology* (1995) 235, 323-337.

Popovich, D.G., PhD, Dierenfeld, E.S., C.N.S., "Gorilla Nutrition". In "Management of Gorillas in Captivity: Husbandry manual, Gorilla Species Survival Plan." Eds. J. Ogden and D. Wharton, American Association of Zoos and Aquariums, 1997.

Popovich, David G., et.al. "The Western Lowland Gorilla Diet Has Implications for the Health of Humans and Other Hominoids," *American Society for Nutritional Sciences*, 1997.

Remis, M.J., Kerr, M.E. "Taste Responses to Fructose and Tannic Acid Among Gorillas (Gorilla gorilla gorilla)," *International Journal of Primatology*, Vol. 23, No. 2, April 2002.

Remis, Melissa J., "Western Lowland Gorillas (Gorilla gorilla gorilla) as Seasonal Frugivores: Use of variable resources," *American Journal of Primatology* 43: 87-109 (1997).

Schaller, George B., *The Mountain Gorilla*, Chicago: University of Chicago Press, 1963.

Schaller, George B., *The Year of the Gorilla*, Chicago: The University of Chicago Press, 1964.

Tutin, Catherine E.G., Fernandez, Michael, "Composition of the Diet of Chimpanzees and Comparisons with that of Sympatric Lowland Gorillas in the Lope Reserve, Gabon," *American Journal of American Primatology*, 30: 195-211 (1993).

Vedder, Amy L. "Movement Patterns of a group of free-Ranging Mountain Gorillas (Gorilla gorilla beringei) and Their relation to Food Availability," *American Journal of Primatology* 7: 73-88 (1984).

Watts, David P. "Composition and Variability of Mountain Gorilla Diets in the Central Virungas," *American Journal of Primatology 7: 323-356 (1984).*

Watts, David P. "Strategies of Habitat Use by Mountain Gorillas," Folia Primatologica, 1991, 56: 1-16.

Watts, David P., "Long-term Habitat Use by Mountain Gorillas (Gorilla gorilla beringei). Reuse of Foraging Areas in Relation to Resource Abundance, Quality and Depletion," *International Journal of Primatology*, Vol. 19, No. 4, 1998.

Watts, David P.,"Long-Term Habitat Use by Mountain Gorillas" (Gorilla gorilla beringei). Consistency, Variation, and home Range Size and Stability," *International Journal Primatology*, Volume 19, No. 4, 1998.

Weber, Bill, Vedder, Amy, *In the Kingdom of Gorillas: The Quest to Save Rwanda's Mountain Gorillas*, London: Aurum Press Ltd., 2002.

Williamson, Elizabeth A., et al., "Composition of the Diet of Lowland Gorillas at Lope in Gabon," *American Journal of Primatology* 21: 265-277 (1990).

Yamagiwa, Juichi, et al., "Seasonal Change in the Composition of the Diet of Eastern Lowland Gorillas," *Primates*, 35 (1): 1-14, January 1994. NB: All references to the Slow Food Movement were found on the Slow Food USA website, www.slowfoodusa.org in 2004.

chapter 5: beyond words

Adams, Reginald, et al., "Effects of Gaze on Amygdala Sensitivity to Anger and Fear Faces," Science, June 6, 2003, vol. 300 p. 1536.

Brody, Marjorie, *Does Your Body Language Stop A Sales Presentation Before It Starts?* Jenkintown, PA: Brody Communications Ltd, 2003.

Brown, William Michael, et. al. "Are there nonverbal cues to commitment? An exploratory study using the zero-acquiantance video presentation paradigm," Evolutionary *Psychology,* 2003. 1:3 42-69.

Bull, Peter, "Nonverbal Communication", *The Psychologist*, Vol. 14, No 12, December 2001.

Darwin, Charles, *The Expressions of the Emotions in Man and Animals*, London: John Murray, 1872.

Dixson, A.F, *The Natural History of the Gorilla*, London: George Weidenfeld and Nicholson, Ltd., 1981.

Ekman, Paul, "Should We Call it Expression of Communication?," *Innovations in Social Science Research*, Vol. 10, No. 4, pp. 333-344, 1997.

Feldman, Robert S. et al., "Nonverbal Deception Abilities and Adolescents' Social Competence: Adolescents with Higher Social Skills are Better Liars," *Journal of Nonverbal Behavior,* 23 (3): 237-249, Fall 1999.

Fossey, Dian, "Vocalizations of the Mountain Gorilla (Gorilla gorilla beringei)," *Animal Behaviour*, 1972, 20, 36-53.

Givens, David B., *The Nonverbal Dictionary of Gestures, Signs & Body Language Cues*, Spokane, Washington: Center for Nonverbal Studies Press, 2004.

Huber, Ernst, *Evolution of the Facial Musculature and Facial Expression*, Baltimore: Johns Hopkins University Press, 1931.

Kendon, Adam, "Gesture", *American Review of Anthropology, 1997, 26: 109-28. 153*

Schaller, George B., *The Mountain Gorilla*, Chicago: University of Chicago Press, 1963.

Tanner, Joanne, E. and Byrne, Richard W. "Concealing Facial evidence of Mood: Perspective-taking in a Captive Gorilla?," *Primates*, 34 (4) 451-457, October 1993.

chapters 6 & 7: gorilla nomenclature and species characteristics & saving the gorilla

"About Gorillas", www.Koko.org/about/facts.html

R Bergin, Patrick, PhD, "Beyond Ebola: Land and Communities Key to Safeguarding Wildlife, African Wildlife Foundation", April 15, 2003.

"Eastern Lowland Gorilla Numbers Plunge to 5,000", National Geographic News.com., March 31, 2004.

"Gorilla in the Midst of Extinction", National Aeronautics and Space Administration, January 6, 2005, www.nasa.gov.

"Gorilla Quick Facts", San Diego Zoo.org.

"Gorillas infecting each other with Ebola", 10 July 2006, newscientist. com news service.

Groves, Jacqueline, "Good News for the Cross River Gorillas?", *Gorilla Journal*, June 2002.

"Hominid Species Timeline," www.wsu.edu.

International Gorilla Conservation programme provided information on companies offering gorilla tours and sound guidelines for visitors using these tours.

Knight, Tim, Gorillas Online, University of Washington, http://staff. washington.edu/timk/gorillas. 155

Lindsley, Tracey, "Gorilla gorilla beringei (Mountain Gorilla)", The University of Michigan, Museum of Zoology, Animal Diversity Web, May 2000.

Meder, Angela, "The genus Gorilla and gorillas in the Wild", 2002.

Millhouse, Christina, "Gorilla gorilla gorilla (Western Lowland Gorilla)", The University of Michigan, Museum of Zoology, Animal Diversity Web, May 2000.

Mountain Gorilla Conservation Fund, www.saveagorilla.org.

Olejniczak, Claudia, "The 21st Century Gorilla: Progress or Perish?," Department of Anthropology, Washington University, Keynote paper, The Apes: Challenges for the 21st Century, Chicago Zoological Society, 2001.

Primates and their Adaptations, www.cartage.org.lb. D

Smithsonian National Zoological Park, "Primates: Gorilla Facts", http://nationalzoo.si.edu.

"Starved by War, Hungry Congolese Turn to Park Animals for Survival", The Associated Press, August 1, 1999.

"The Living Africa, Gorilla: Gorilla gorilla", Thinkquest Team, 1998 (http://library.thinkquest.org).

Warren, Adrian, "Mountain Gorillas", www.lastrefuge.co.uk.

WWF and Gorillas, World Wild Fund, www.worldwildlife.org/gorillas. www.bergorilla.de (includes research and estimates on populations and effects of Ebola, among a broad range of other issues).

www.Wikipedia.com.
www.yorku.ca/gibeault/gorillas.html.

index

about the author

Andrew Grant has served as Deputy Director of the San Diego Zoo and Wild Animal Park and Managing Director of The London Zoo. Grant has also held executive positions at Busch Gardens and Universal Studios Tours. Through his involvement with these institutions, he worked with some of the world's most pre-eminent zoologists, conservationists, and primatologists. Grant's ongoing fascination with primates, and, specifically, the gorilla subspecies, formed the inspiration for *Rain Forest Wisdom*. He has appeared as an expert witness on numerous projects in the United States and overseas. He currently lives in Santa Barbara, CA.

about the illustrator

Zach Horvath is an award-winning Brooklyn, NY, based artist specializing in illustration and fine arts. He is currently working as a designer for s.b.art.design and is illustrating several upcoming children's picture books.